FAITHFUL WARRIOR

FAITHFUL WARRIOR

Praying with HOPE for Women Battling Cancer

Katherine Hedlund

NEW YORK

FAITHFUL WARRIOR

Praying with HOPE for Women Battling Cancer

Published in New York, New York, by Morgan James Publishing. Morgan James and The Entrepreneurial Publisher are trademarks of Morgan James, LLC.
www.MorganJamesPublishing.com

The Morgan James Speakers Group can bring authors to your live event. For more information or to book an event visit The Morgan James Speakers Group at
www.TheMorganJamesSpeakersGroup.com.

All Scripture quotations, unless otherwise indicated, are taken from the Holy Bible, New International Version®, NIV®, copyright ©1973, 1978, 1984 by Biblica, Inc.™ Used by permission of Zondervan. All rights reserved worldwide. www.zondervan.com The "NIV" and "New International Version" are trademarks registered in the United States Patent and Trademark Office by Biblica, Inc.™

Scripture quotations marked NASB are taken from the New American Standard Bible®, copyright © 1960, 1962, 1963, 1968, 1971, 1972, 1973, 1975, 1977, 1995 by The Lockman Foundation. Used by permission. (www.Lockman.org)

Scripture quotations marked AMP are taken from the Amplified Bible, copyright © 1954, 1958, 1962, 1964, 1965, 1987 by The Lockman Foundation. Used by permission.

Scripture quotations marked NLT are taken from the Holy Bible, New Living Translation, copyright © 1996, 2004, 2007 by Tyndale House Foundation. Used by permission of Tyndale House Publishers, Inc., Carol Stream, Illinois 60188. All rights reserved.

Scripture quotations from *THE MESSAGE*, copyright © by Eugene H Peterson 1993, 1994, 1995, 1996, 2000, 2001, 2002. Used by permission of NavPress Publishing Group.

A FREE eBook edition is available
with the purchase of this print book

CLEARLY PRINT YOUR NAME IN THE BOX ABOVE

Instructions to claim your free eBook edition:
1. Download the BitLit app for Android or iOS
2. Write your name in UPPER CASE in the box
3. Use the BitLit app to submit a photo
4. Download your eBook to any device

ISBN 978-1-61448-934-4 paperback
ISBN 978-1-61448-935-1 eBook
ISBN 978-1-61448-936-8 audio
ISBN 978-1-61448-937-5 hardcover
Library of Congress Control Number:
2013951454

Cover Design by:
Chris Treccani
www.3dogdesign.net

Interior Design by:
Bonnie Bushman
bonnie@caboodlegraphics.com

In an effort to support local communities, raise awareness and funds, Morgan James Publishing donates a percentage of all book sales for the life of each book to Habitat for Humanity Peninsula and Greater Williamsburg.

Get involved today, visit
www.MorganJamesBuilds.com

Habitat
for Humanity®
Peninsula and
Greater Williamsburg
Building Partner

To Linda Carter, who prompted these prayers.
To Bridget Valko, who kept the prayers flowing.
I am honored to have soldiered with you in your fight.
You are both so very brave.

Table of Contents

Foreword

My friendship with Katherine Hedlund bloomed on Christmas Day, 2006, on the one-year anniversary of my husband's death. She presented me with a gift unlike any I'd ever received.

After twelve months Kat, as friends call her, handed me a prayer journal she wrote and kept especially for my sons and me during our most painful season of grief.

I had no idea Katherine was keeping this journal for us, so when I began reading it a flood of emotion washed over me. The words "I'll pray for you" meant something very real. In our darkest hours my friend was quietly interceding on our behalf to restore us. Isn't that just how the Spirit works?

> *"We do not know what we ought to pray for, but the Spirit himself intercedes for us through wordless groans. And he who searches our hearts knows the mind of the Spirit, because the Spirit intercedes for God's people in accordance with the will of God."*
> *Romans 8:26-27*

When we could not pray for ourselves, the Spirit led Katherine to pray relentlessly for us. Looking back, it's clear that our lives were a reflection of the peace and power of those prayers. Each of us has the ability to give the gift of prayer, and now there is a book that can help you use that gift to help others.

When Kat told me she was writing *Faithful Warrior*, I was overjoyed. This book is a vital companion for the journey of cancer. Her prayers become your prayers. She reaches into your heart and gives voice to the agony and helplessness you feel when a loved one is suffering. The prayers will draw you closer to God, awaken the Holy Spirit in you and empower you to be a prayer warrior on behalf of a loved one battling cancer.

Katherine's beautiful insight, personal experience with cancer (she too is a survivor!), and utter reliance on the Word of God will be an invaluable resource and comfort for caregivers, patients, and supportive friends and family members far and wide.

I pray this book is the beginning of your friendship with Kat and that her words, filled with God-breathed Scripture and personal reflections, will guide and give you strength as you sojourn with a loved one through the bittersweet agony of cancer.

—Gina Kell Spehn
Author of *New York Times* bestseller *The Color of Rain*
Executive Director, New Day Foundation for Families

My HOPE Bird

Have you ever thought that HOPE has a color? Well, I have. I tend to put visual tags on things and often relate them to nature. For me, HOPE is a vibrant red Cardinal. If you live, or have ever lived, anywhere that winter is harsh and often shrouded in snow, you can certainly understand my choice of this brilliant little bird.

When winter is cold, dark and bleak, the appearance of a bright red Cardinal resting on a snow-laden bough is something that absolutely thrills my soul. I find myself searching for him... listening for his song. When I see my scarlet friend flying from branch to branch it's as if God is reminding me that He's still there, still in control and still the God of HOPE. So I keep watching and waiting for this little bird to appear.

When I'm washing dishes by the kitchen window, I keep glancing up to see if I can catch a flicker of his ruby-brightness on the stripped-bare branches. When I'm going out to get the mail, I stop for a few chilly moments to listen for his trilling melody. Oh, that I would always set my heart to be in search of the God of HOPE with the same anticipation and expectation.

Winter, whether a calendar season or a season in your heart, will eventually give way to spring, and there will be fresh new growth again. You can count on it. You can trust in it. You can look forward to it. Even now. Even in this. There is always HOPE.

And we rejoice in the hope of the glory of God. Not only so, but we also rejoice in our sufferings, because we know that suffering produces perseverance; perseverance, character; and character, hope. And hope does not disappoint us, because God has poured out his love into our hearts by the Holy Spirit, whom he has given us.
Romans 5:2-5

Preface

Cancer. You hear the word. Your heart stops. Unfair. Frightening. Life. Death. Whether the diagnosis is yours or that of a precious friend or loved one, the question is always the same, How can I fight this overwhelming disease? You can't. Not really. But God can.

> *The Lord is my light and my salvation—of whom shall I fear?*
>
> *The Lord is the stronghold of my life—of whom shall I be afraid? Though an army besiege me, my heart will not fear, though war break out against me, even then will I be confident. One thing I ask of the Lord, this is what I seek: that I may dwell in the house of the Lord all the days of my life, to gaze upon the beauty of the Lord and to seek him in his temple. For in the day of trouble he will keep me safe in his dwelling; he will hide me in the shelter of his tabernacle and set me high upon a rock*
>
> *Psalm 27:1, 3-5*

January 17, 2000, ushered in the crushing blow. Kind eyes delivering cruel words. "You have cancer and that sucks, but yours is the very best kind." Is there such a thing? All these survival-years later I grin at the thought.

Cancer is mind-numbing. I would arrive at a destination and not remember how I got there...read a book for hours without any idea who the characters were...lie awake at night and wonder what my life would be like...wonder if there would even be a life.

Fragmented, scattered thoughts traipsed across my mind. How could I help myself when I couldn't even keep track of the days?

I lift up my eyes to the hills—where does my help come from? My help comes from the Lord, the Maker of heaven and earth.

He will not let your foot slip—he who watches over you will not slumber...The Lord watches over you—the Lord is your shade at your right hand; the sun will not harm you by day, nor the moon by night. The Lord will keep you from all harm—he will watch over your life; the Lord will watch over your coming and going both now and forever more.

Psalm 121

Here was my answer. Here is yours.

Whether you are fighting for your own life or the life of another, the battle starts here. Each prayer has a place to insert a name, personalizing it to fit your situation. It is my hope that these simple, Scripture-based prayers give you the words and strength you need to wage war on this illness, no matter what form it takes or whom it has attacked.

Many times I couldn't understand why I was doing so well. How could I have peace in the midst of disease-filled turmoil? How could I face each new treatment with hope? The answer is both simple and wildly complex. It was because of prayer.

Through your faithful prayers and the generous response of the Spirit of Jesus Christ, everything he wants to do in and through me will be done.
Philippians 1:19

I truly believe it was the prayers of the Faithful Warriors in my life that sustained me through the darkest days, their petitions lifting me to the throne of grace.

To each and every one of them I raise my sword.

Acknowledgments

Many tears were shed during the writing of this book. Not out of frustration, mind you, but out of sheer, overwhelming gratitude. There were times when I was writing these prayers that I just had to stop and cry. As tears rolled down my cheeks, I marveled, once again, that God had spared my life. My life has never been more important or valuable than the lives that have been lost to this disease. Nor do my family and friends love me more deeply than the family and friends who have been left behind with only their memories.

There are many things that I will never know about my cancer journey, but what I *do* know is that it was *all grace* that kept me here…just as it would have been *all grace* if the outcome had been different. All grace. All goodness. All God. I have barely begun to scratch the surface of how amazing that truly is.

To my family and friends

If you've prayed for me during my time of cancer or lung "mysteries" (remember that?), heartache or joy, indecision or exciting new adventures (such as the writing of this book), then

xvi

you are one of my Faithful Warriors. I rely on you more than you know. I am more grateful than mere words can express.

To my husband, Gary

Behind every creative woman is a patient, supportive man. You are both of those things and so much more. Whether it's listening to more than thirty years of student piano recitals, cleaning the bathroom when I'm in the middle of this deadline or picking up dinner because a "home cooked meal" just wasn't on my radar, you patiently supported me. *That* is your love language, "Herman". Thank you for speaking it so eloquently over my life throughout the years.

To my son, Eric

You were my first joy and continue to make my heart smile. The cover design concept is exactly what I was hoping for. Thanks so much for getting the whole thing rolling. Your creativity amazes me. Crafting words, creating music or capturing a slice of life on canvas, your giftedness is something I greatly appreciate. I'll always be your biggest fan, but you already know that.

To my daughter, Holly

No daughter could be better, and no mama could be more blessed! Thank you so much for preparing the manuscript. What would have been a computer nightmare for me was a piece of cake for you. What a relief! You are the bright spot of every day and the delight of my heart. Whether running for food in Chicago, laughing hysterically over who-knows-what or simply hanging out, our time together is always the best. You know, I was always a bit afraid of having a girl…but if they were all like you, my Sweetie Bean, I would have had a dozen. Loves you!

To my son-in-law, Bryce
   One of the pages in your wedding scrapbook says, *"We just enlarged our home by 6 feet, 4 inches."* Best addition we ever made! For twenty-three years I was the mother of two, but I have to say, having you for a son has more than tripled the fun and the joy. I couldn't love or appreciate you more.

To my Love-Love, Austin
   Everyone told me how much I'd love being a grandparent, but I had no clue how wonderful it would be until you were born. Spending time with you, seeing the world through your eyes and watching you grow…that is what I call happiness. Who needs a "bucket list" when their bucket is already overflowing! I love being your Mimi!

To our soon-to-arrive grandbaby
   At the completion of this book, we are anxiously awaiting your arrival. I know you'll be precious, just like your big brother. I know you'll be loved up to the moon and back. But, what I don't know is…should I buy blue or pink? You are the best surprise, Little One! I can't wait to meet you!

To my editor extraordinaire, Carolyn Pruitt
   Sissy. Honsey. Bestie. Each of those names means the world to me. So many years and so many miles, yet we still share the same heart. You know me inside-out. You know how I think,

write, live and love. Who else could have been my editor? Who else would have made sure this turned out exactly the way I had envisioned it? Who else could have been my "Happi"? You, my dear, sweet friend, are the most faithful of warriors. How I loved sharing this wild, e-coupon ride with you.

To Morgan James Publishing

Giving birth to a book is hard work. How grateful I am to my team at MJP for coaching me throughout this process and reminding me to breathe.

To my Redeemer, Savior, Friend

How You can take this fragile, cracked vessel and make it worthy for Your good purpose will never cease to amaze me. Thank You, Jesus, for being the Author and Finisher of my faith. You are the One who writes the best stories ever!

Last, but not least, to you, dear reader

I'm sorry you had to buy this book because it means that someone you love is hurting. How I pray that these God-infused words will fill you with peace, courage, and hope. If my diagnosis of cancer helps just one person, the journey was worth it.

Preparing for War

Prayers after Cancer Diagnosis

As for God, his way is perfect...He is a shield for all who take refuge in him. For who is God besides the Lord? And who is the Rock except our God? It is God who arms me with strength and makes my way perfect...He trains my hands for battle; my arms can bend a bow of bronze. You give me your shield of victory and your right hand sustains me.

Psalm 18:30-32, 34, 35

To the cancer patient

How can this be? Hearing the diagnosis of cancer is enough to stop you in your tracks, sending a cold wave of fear throughout your entire being. Who would enlist for this? Certainly not you. Denial and anger are twin emotions flowing through your mind and heart right now. Now is the time to call on those who will share this fight with you. Now is the time to ready yourself for the battle ahead. And so it begins.

To the Faithful Warrior

Now is the time to put on your armor.

Though a host encamp against me, my heart shall not fear; though war arise against me, yet I will be confident.

Psalm 27:3

Today, Lord, I pray for a deep steadiness in _____'s heart, soul, mind and spirit. Cancer has "encamped" itself against her. It has ambushed her and attacked her. It has caused her entire world to shake on its foundation. Though it rises against her, Lord, YOU rise higher!

Build a deep abiding trust within her heart-of-hearts. Everything about this part of her life-journey is scary and unknown, but I pray You would strengthen her to respond in trust.

God, please just reach down to take hold of her hand and lead her down this boulder-strewn path. You know the dangers and pitfalls of her treatment. You know the loneliness of wrestling with this diagnosis in the middle of the night. You know the deep longing to have this "cup" taken from her.

In all these things, please draw close to her. Assure her and her family of Your abiding, steadfast, everlasting love. Remind them throughout this day that Your thoughts are always rushing toward them and Your riches are unsearchable.

Yes, I have loved you with an everlasting love;
therefore with loving-kindness have I drawn you
and continued My faithfulness to you.
Jeremiah 31:3 (AMP)

And I pray that you, being rooted and established in love,
may have power, together with all the saints, to grasp how
wide and long and high and deep is the love of Christ, and
to know this love that surpasses knowledge—that you may be
filled to the measure of all the fullness of God.
Ephesians 3:17-19

A Note of HOPE

_____

_____

_____

_____

_____

_____

_____

_____

_____

In your distress you called and I rescued you, I
answered you out of a thundercloud.
Psalm 81:7

Father God,

The weight of this diagnosis feels like the gathering and
building of a great thundercloud. The sky is becoming dark…
ominous…threatening. We look up and see it moving, but there's
nothing we can do to hold it back.

I ask You to speak to _____ from the center of this impending
storm. She needs You so much right now, Lord. Calm her fears
and quiet her mind, settling the turbulence she's feeling. We
always hear about "the calm before the storm," but today I pray
for "the calm *within* the storm."

Be her steadiness. I know her thoughts are still reeling from
this diagnosis, so I simply ask You to gather them together and
give her the wisdom and discernment she needs for the difficult
decisions that are ahead of her.

Please be gracious to her family. Wrap them in Your tender
care as they hunker down alongside her to weather this frightening
storm. Denial might seem pretty attractive at this point in time,
but I pray You would help them face the reality of this situation
with strength and grace.

None of us can do this without You, Lord, so please stay closer
than the very air that surrounds each of us.

O LORD, I have come to You for protection; don't let me be disgraced. Save me, for You do what is right. Turn Your ear to listen to me; rescue me quickly. Be my rock of protection, a fortress where I will be safe. You are my rock and my fortress. For the honor of Your name, lead me out of this danger. Pull me from the trap my enemies set for me, for I find protection in You alone. I entrust my spirit into Your hand. Rescue me LORD, for You are a faithful God.
Psalm 31:1-5 (NLT)

If any of you is deficient in wisdom, let him ask of the giving God [Who gives] to everyone liberally and ungrudgingly, without reproaching or faultfinding, and it will be given him.
James 1:5 (AMP)

A Note of HOPE

_____

_____

_____

_____

_____

_____

_____

_____

_____

_____

I'm not trying to get my way in the world's way.
I'm trying to get Your way, Your Word's way.
I'm staying on the trail; I'm putting one foot in
front of the other. I'm not giving up.
Psalm 17:4, 5 (THE MESSAGE)

Father God,

Again I lift _____ to You. I place her in Your loving and gracious hands and ask You to do Your perfect will in her life. For *all* the things going on in her personal world, I pray this powerful verse.

I pray that she would not try to get her way, make her way or find her way according to the world and all its "definitions." Instead, may she understand and discern Your perfect way for her as she reads Your Word and talks with You.

In the midst of everything that's going on in her heart and mind, I pray You would keep her walking steadily down the path of Your uniquely designed purpose for her life. Though her path is unfamiliar, You have promised to be her guide.

As I think about _____, I think about all the changes that are happening. We don't like change, and so often we fight against it. How I pray for her to *lean into* the change, instead of *pushing away* from it. Strengthen her to look at it, listen to it, absorb it and embrace it. What a beautifully hard road she's traveling.

I will lead the blind by ways they have not known, along unfamiliar paths I will guide them; I will turn the darkness into light before them and make the rough places smooth. These are the things I will do; I will not forsake them.
Isaiah 42:16

Do not be conformed to this world (this age), [fashioned after and adapted to its external, superficial customs], but be transformed (changed) by the [entire] renewal of your mind [by its new ideals and its new attitude], so that you may prove [for yourselves] what is the good and acceptable and perfect will of God, even the thing which is good and acceptable and perfect [in His sight for you].
Romans 12:2 (AMP)

A Note of HOPE

For I know the plans I have for you, declares the
Lord, plans to prosper you and not harm you,
plans to give you hope and a future.
Jeremiah 29:11

Dear Lord,

I know You have wonderful plans for _____. Plans with a future, a hope, a path of goodness. How I pray You will strengthen her and assure her for what lies ahead, whether it is known or unknown.

This diagnosis, Lord, it wasn't planned for or hoped for, so how can we refer to it as "a path of goodness?" These are the things we will probably never understand. But we *do* know that nothing can touch us without Your permission. Again I'm baffled by that thought.

Lord, in the shock of this course-altering event, I ask You to remind _____, deep within her being, that if You've called her to do something then You will most assuredly be there too! You don't ask her to go through this alone. You don't leave her unprepared. You don't stand aside and watch. You enter in. You engage. You show her *Emmanuel*...God with us.

Blaze this truth upon her shaken heart. Build her inner strength and confidence. Let her fully commit to her personal preparation for the battle ahead. War has been declared.

As for God, his way is perfect:
The Lord's word is flawless;
He shields all who take refuge in him.
For who is God besides the Lord?
And who is the Rock except our God?
It is God who arms me with strength
and keeps my way secure.
Psalm 18:30-32

Casting the whole of your care [all your anxieties, all your
worries, all your concerns, once and for all] on Him, for He
cares for you affectionately and cares about you watchfully.
1 Peter 5:7 (AMP)

A Note of HOPE

_____

_____

_____

_____

_____

_____

_____

_____

_____

_____

"You will conquer. Do not fear changes. You can never fear changes when I, your Lord, change not. Jesus Christ, the same yesterday, today and forever. I am beside you. Steadfastness, unchangingness, come to you, too, as you dwell in Me. Rest in Me."
From *God Calling* by Arthur J. Russell

Father, may _____ gain a sense of conquering as she enters into this unwanted phase of her life. In the midst of all this change, I praise You for Your unchanging nature. Thank You for remaining as the *only* true steadiness in our out-of-balance world.

So often we feel defeated by life, with no glimpse of victory in sight. But You have promised that we are *more* than conquerors through You, the Unchanging One!

Lord, I ask You to take hold of _____'s hand as she steps out into "The Great Unknown." Dispel her fear and replace it with the anticipation of Your blessings.

May she rest in the fact that You are beside her all the way. You don't miss a turn. You don't skip a step. You aren't surprised by a change of pace. Nothing catches You unaware because You've already gone before her on this journey. Your Word says that You take great delight in her, longing to be the quiet, calming presence in her heart, soul, mind and spirit. May it be so, dear Lord.

The Lord your God is with you,
the Mighty Warrior who saves.
He will take great delight in you;
in his love he will no longer rebuke you,
but will rejoice over you with singing.
Zephaniah 3:17

Yet amid all these things we are more than conquerors and
gain a surpassing victory through Him Who loved us.
Romans 8:37 (AMP)

A Note of HOPE

_____
_____
_____
_____
_____
_____
_____
_____
_____

Bless the Lord, oh my soul, and all that is within
me, bless his holy name.
Psalm 103:1

O Lord,

May we be turned inside-out with blessing and thankfulness. In the hard places of physical and emotional pain, I pray You would teach us to make the decision to bless Your holy name.

I'm still shaking my head at the hard truth of this quote by C.S. Lewis: *"If you think of the world as a place intended simply for our happiness, you find it quite intolerable. Think of it as a place of training and correction, and it's not so bad."*

Lord, strengthen and equip _____to bless Your name as she lifts up prayers of thankfulness in the midst of the devastating places of life. Give her eyes to see You at work and ears to hear Your sweet, soothing voice. Speak to her frightened heart in a language that only she understands.

Wrap her up tightly in Your arms today. Questions concerning her upcoming treatment are undoubtedly rolling around in her mind. Please steady the mental "tossing and turning," keeping her firmly grounded in You.

Enter into His gates with thanksgiving and a thank offering and into His courts with praise! Be thankful and say so to Him, bless and affectionately praise His name! For the Lord is good; His mercy and loving-kindness are everlasting, His faithfulness and truth endure to all generations.
Psalm 100:4, 5 (AMP)

If you don't know what you're doing, pray to the Father. He loves to help. You'll get His help and won't be condescended to when you ask for it. Ask boldly, believingly, without a second thought. People who "worry their prayers" are like wind-whipped waves.
James 1:5-7 (THE MESSAGE)

A Note of HOPE

_____

_____

_____

_____

_____

_____

_____

_____

_____

_____

_____

The Lord is close to the brokenhearted and saves
those who are crushed in spirit.
Psalm 34:18

Dear Lord,

I'm not sure if the shock of this diagnosis has lessened yet. Probably not. If *my* mind is numb, I can only imagine what _____ is feeling. How grateful I am that You know her completely. You know exactly what is going on in her mind and heart right now, and You're the only One who can truly minister to her in that place of uncertainty and fear.

You promised You would be close to the brokenhearted and the crushed in spirit. I'm holding You to that, Lord. I ask You to weave Your beautiful blessings throughout her life today. Give her a reason to smile and an awareness of Your nearness.

Strengthen her in the midst of all that is devastating and enable her to *choose joy*. May she be a woman of thankfulness despite the detours that have come into her life. There are so many questions, Lord, and not nearly enough answers. Help her to wait patiently. Help her to wait trustingly. Help her to wait expectantly for all that is ahead of her. As the saying goes, *"I do not know what the future holds, but I know Who holds the future."* May she firmly tether her life to that truth in a deeper, richer way.

I will extol the Lord at all times; his praise will always be on my lips. My soul will boast in the Lord; let the afflicted hear and rejoice. Glorify the Lord with me; let us exalt his name together.
Psalm 34:1-3

Through Him, therefore, let us constantly and at all times offer up to God a sacrifice of praise, which is the fruit of lips that thankfully acknowledge and confess and glorify His name.
Hebrews 13:15 (AMP)

A Note of HOPE

_____

_____

_____

_____

_____

_____

_____

_____

_____

_____

Be joyful in hope, patient in affliction, faithful in prayer.
Romans 12:12

That's it, Lord. These three exhortations are what we need on a daily, moment-by-moment basis.

You've told us to rejoice in You always, to look at each day as a hand-crafted gift from You and to shout out the glories that are Yours and Yours alone.

I pray these very things for _____today. Please give her wonderful reasons to *rejoice*. Let her see You in the unfolding story proclaimed in the sunrise, weaving its wonderful narration all the way to the setting of the sun.

So often we fly through our day without taking any notice of the hand-crafted gifts that surround us. The delicacy of a flower... the dimples on a baby's hand...the happy chirping of a brightly feathered bird. It's all from Your hand. All for us to enjoy. How I pray _____would look at her world today, peeking around corners to see You at work and digging deep to find treasures buried deep.

May delightful thoughts be on her mind and joyous words be on her lips. This is the day You have made, Lord, and that means it's a great day to be glad!

From the rising of the sun to the place where it sets,
the name of the Lord is to be praised.
Psalm 113:3

Celebrate God all day, every day. I mean, revel in Him!
Philippians 4:4 (THE MESSAGE)

A Note of HOPE

_____

_____

_____

_____

_____

_____

_____

_____

_____

_____

e me produce.

"When any troubled soul fails to see that God is enough, I feel like saying, not with scorn but with infinite care, 'Ah, dear friend, you do not know God! If you knew Him you could not help seeing that He is the remedy for every need of your soul.'"
From God Is Enough by Hannah Whitall Smith

What beautiful truths written here, Lord. May _____ see You as "the remedy for every need of her soul." May she rely on You through every moment, every thought, every step of this journey.

Father, how I pray she would be fully grounded in *You*. Let her send down roots of faith and assurance that are strong and deep, roots that remain firm no matter how the storm is raging above ground.

Bring a kaleidoscope of friends to her side. Some to encourage her, some to laugh with her, some to cry with her, some to pray with her and some to eat chocolate with her! She will need a full spectrum of friends along this road.

And she will need You, Lord, as her closest and dearest Friend. Always there to steady her when life just feels overly wobbly and uncertain. Always there to hold her tight with both gentleness and grace. Always. There.

Rejoice with those who rejoice [sharing others' joy], and weep with those who weep [sharing others' grief].
Romans 12:15 (AMP)

Energize the limp hands, strengthen the rubbery knees.
Tell the fearful souls, "Courage! Take heart! God is here,
right here, on His way to put things right and
redress all wrongs. He's on His Way! He'll save you!"
Isaiah 35:3, 4 (THE MESSAGE)

A Note of HOPE

_____

_____

_____

_____

_____

_____

_____

_____

_____

_____

> *LORD, you are my God; I will exalt you and praise your name, for in perfect faithfulness you have done wonderful things, things planned long ago... You have been a refuge for the poor, a refuge for the needy in his distress, a shelter from the storm and a shade from the heat. For the breath of the ruthless is like a storm driving against a wall.*
>
> *Isaiah 25:1, 4*

Perfect faithfulness. What more could we ask for, Lord? I know we would like easy or exciting or fun, but would that really be the best for us? Probably not, even though it might feel better!

Lord, You do all things in perfect faithfulness. It's not selective. It's not random. It's not hit or miss. And not only is everything done in *perfect faithfulness*, but You say they're *marvelous* things—things You planned (in perfect faithfulness) so long ago. I wrestle with this, Lord.

I look at _____, and it's hard for me to think her cancer is part of Your perfect faithfulness. Where is the marvelous in all of this? I believe You are in control and You are using this to further refine her life; yet how I wish her journey had taken a different path.

For all that is hard in her situation, You've promised to be a Refuge and Shelter. May this ruthless disease find itself driving up against a wall—a wall of perfectly faithful healing and grace. Please, Lord, please!

God is a safe place to hide,
ready to help when we need Him.
We stand fearless at the cliff-edge of doom,
courageous in seastorm and earthquake,
Before the rush and roar of oceans,
the tremors that shift mountains.
Psalm 46:1-3 (THE MESSAGE)

And the God of all grace, who called you to his eternal glory
in Christ, after you have suffered a little while,
will himself restore you and make you strong, firm and
steadfast. To him be the power for ever and ever. Amen.
1 Peter 5:10-11

A Note of HOPE

_____

_____

_____

_____

_____

_____

_____

_____

_____

_____

But I trusted in, relied on, and was confident in You, O Lord; I said, You are my God. My times are in Your hands; deliver me from the hands of my foes and those who pursue me and persecute me. Let Your face shine on Your servant; save me for Your mercy's sake and in Your loving-kindness.

Psalm 31:14-16 (AMP)

I *know* You have _____'s future in Your hands.
I *know* You cause all things to work together for good.
I *know* You rush Your mercies to her every morning.
I *know* You are always thinking about her.
I *know* You have counted the number of hairs on her head.
I *know* You will guide and direct her along unfamiliar paths.
I *know* You love her with an everlasting love.
I *know* You will steady her with Your perfect peace.
I *know* You have drawn her with loving-kindness.
I *know* nothing is impossible with You.
I *know* You fight her battle.
I *know* You carry her burdens.
I *know* You care for her…truly…deeply.

All these things I know, dear Lord. Now I ask You to speak all these truths to _____'s heart and spirit. May every fiber of her being absorb these magnificent things and, by heavenly "osmosis," be strengthened and changed forever and daily by them.

Ah, Sovereign LORD, you have made the
heavens and the earth by your great power and
outstretched arm. Nothing is too hard for you.
Jeremiah 32:17

Therefore we do not become discouraged (utterly spiritless,
exhausted, and wearied out through fear). Though our outer
man is [progressively] decaying and wasting away, yet our
inner self is being [progressively] renewed day after day.
2 Corinthians 4:16 (AMP)

A Note of HOPE

_____

_____

_____

_____

_____

_____

_____

_____

_____

_____

> *Send forth your light and truth, let them guide*
> *me...Put your hope in God, for I will yet praise*
> *him, my Savior and my God.*
> **Psalm 43:3, 5**

Dear Jesus,

Strengthen _____'s heart to trust in Your ever-constant love for her. May she sense Your presence and care in ways far beyond her comprehension, knowing You will meet her every need in ways she could never even imagine.

Give her truth and light each day, guiding her steps and her thoughts. May she find safe refuge in You as she finds Your name on her lips, giving praise in the midst of the difficult and confusing.

It is in Your powerful and matchless name that I pray for _____today. Let all things bright and beautiful be upon her life. Let all things hopeful and helpful fill her mind. Dispel the darkness and doubt, enabling her to dwell in Your perfect peace.

She is facing many changes ahead. Changes to her body, her routine, her outlook, her plans, her priorities, her *everything*. Keep developing her trust "muscles" as she walks this oh-so-hard path. You are before her. You are behind her. You are beside her all the way. I know this with absolute certainty because You promised!

May her life with You be richer and fuller because of this unwelcome detour.

*I look behind me and You're there,
then up ahead and You're there, too—
Your reassuring presence, coming and going.
This is too much, too wonderful—
I can't take it all in!
Psalm 139:5, 6 (THE MESSAGE)*

*When it was evening, the boat was in the middle of
the sea, and He was alone on the land. Seeing them
straining at the oars, for the wind was against them,
at about the fourth watch of the night He came to
them, walking on the sea; and He intended to pass by
them. But when they saw Him walking on the sea, they
supposed that it was a ghost, and cried out; for they all
saw Him and were terrified. But immediately He spoke
with them and said to them, "Take courage; it is I, do
not be afraid." Then He got into the boat with them,
and the wind stopped; and they were utterly astonished.
Mark 6:47-51 (NASB)*

A Note of HOPE

_____
_____
_____
_____
_____
_____

How long, LORD? Will you forget me forever?
How long must I wrestle with my thoughts and
day after day have sorrow in my heart? How
long will my enemy triumph over me?
Psalm 13:1-2

I know _____can fully relate to the psalmist David when he penned these words. How could she not! An enemy is working to triumph over her, defeat her. Don't let it, God! I know You are constantly watching over her and rushing Your love toward her. I know she is always on Your mind, just as I am. Help her to keep her thoughts centered on You rather than giving in to this very real fear. I need that too, Lord, for my mind is running off in scattered directions even as I'm praying this right now.

What _____is living through right now is overwhelming, but it's also overwhelming to those of us who love her. Father, spread Your perfect peace over every character in this story. Each one of us needs You in a different way, so I ask You to mercifully tailor Your comfort and guidance to meet each of those individual needs.

How grateful I am that You are a personal God. Never standing off in the distance, but remaining just a thought's breath away.

How precious to me are your thoughts, God!
How vast is the sum of them!
Were I to count them,
they would outnumber the grains of sand—
when I awake, I am still with you.
Psalm 139:17, 18

And my God will liberally supply (fill to the full) your every
need according to His riches in glory in Christ Jesus.
Philippians 4:19 (AMP)

A Note of HOPE

_____

_____

_____

_____

_____

_____

_____

_____

_____

_____

By wisdom a house is built, and by understanding it is established; through knowledge its rooms are filled with rare and beautiful treasures.
Proverbs 24:3-4

We're always building our "house" no matter what stage of life we're in. There are very few times when "construction" ceases since You always seem to have plans for "remodeling" in the works!

Lord, as _____ continues to build her house, I ask You to impart wisdom, understanding and knowledge. Guide her through the difficult decisions and then give her the courage to make them. Escort her to a place of complete stability in all areas of her life: emotional, physical, spiritual, relational and financial.

How I pray she would wake each morning and simply breathe You in. May she surrender all that causes her anxiety and worry. I ask You to be the voice of calm in her head, the steadying hand on her shoulder and her warm covering of peace—the peace that passes all understanding and trumps every one of her circumstances.

The reality of building our house never lets up. How grateful I am that in the never-letting-up You never let us go!

The Lord is my Shepherd [to feed, guide, and shield me], I shall not lack. He makes me lie down in [fresh, tender] green pastures; He leads me beside the still and restful waters. He refreshes and restores my life (myself); He leads me in the paths of righteousness [uprightness and right standing with Him—not for my earning it, but] for His name's sake.
Psalm 23:1-3 (AMP)

Peace I leave with you; my peace I give you.
I do not give to you as the world gives.
Do not let your hearts be troubled and do not be afraid.
John 14:27

A Note of HOPE

_____

_____

_____

_____

_____

_____

_____

_____

_____

And God is able to bless you abundantly, so that in all things at all times, having all that you need, you will abound in every good work.
2 Corinthians 9:8

O Lord,

This verse brings a smile to my heart. It overflows with hope and assurance and the blessed goodness of who You are.

Able. Abundantly. All. Abound. These are such wonderful words of encouragement for a time when things appear so discouraging.

Please release Your abundant ability into _____'s life. Let her sense that *"all things at all times"* are being covered by You. Nothing will fall short. Nothing will be overlooked. Nothing will be deemed unimportant. You have promised to provide her with everything she needs so she can flourish and grow and *"abound in every good work."*

The idea of having cancer and abounding in good works seems contradictory, Lord, but that's where You step in. When she gives a smile or an encouraging word, when she lends a listening ear or utters a fervent prayer, when she shares a tear with another hurting cancer sufferer—all these things can be abounding evidence of *Your* work in *her* good works. Father God, please give her an assortment of divine opportunities to be Your hands, Your words and Your heart. Give her an abundance of strength and grace to share with those around her who are struggling. May she bring light and hope to others while in the midst of her own dark and difficult circumstances.

Have mercy on me, Lord, for I call to you all day long. Bring joy to your servant, Lord, for I put my trust in you. You, Lord, are forgiving and good, abounding in love to all who call to you.
Psalm 86:3-5

Now all glory to God, who is able, through His mighty power at work within us, to accomplish infinitely more than we might ask or think.
Ephesians 3:20 (NLT)

A Note of HOPE

And without faith it is impossible to please God,
because anyone who comes to him must believe
that he exists and that he rewards those who
earnestly seek him.
Hebrews 11:6

Dear Lord,

This *set apart* time for _____ is such a beautiful, ripe opportunity for her to please You! What a *faith* it takes to walk day after day without knowing why You have allowed this. What a *faith* it takes to hang on to You for her full and complete healing. What a *faith* it takes for her to realize this could be the most pleasing year of her life.

The message of this scripture is almost too upside-down to fathom! How could she please You when her body is ravaged with cancer? How could she delight Your heart when treatment leaves her physically and emotionally depleted? How, Lord? How can it be?

By faith.

Lord, may she earnestly, diligently, faithfully, joyfully seek You. And may You lavishly, abundantly, graciously, miraculously reward her. What a legacy of faith and faithfulness You are building *in* her life and *through* her life.

Bless her today, Lord. Boost her spirits and touch her heart with Your abiding and loving presence. Surprise her with an extra helping of joy. As she walks "by faith" she is fulfilling her calling.

If you do not stand firm in your faith,
you will not stand at all.
Isaiah 7:9

For we live by faith, not by sight.
2 Corinthians 5:7

A Note of HOPE

For God so loved the world, that He gave His only begotten Son, that whoever believes in Him shall not perish, but have eternal life.
John 3:16 (NASB)

Lord God,

You said that You live within the praises of Your people, at home and settled down. That is a miraculous thought, God. I look at this life, how *unsettling* it is, and I wonder *how* You can do it. *Why* You would do it. But then it always comes back to the love. The love You have for us is beyond measure. I stand amazed and grateful for the millionth time.

Today I simply want to praise You. Today I simply want to speak out who You are in our lives. Today I simply want to experience the tremendous security of Your very character and nature.

You are our *Light* and our *Hope.*
You are our *Shepherd* and our *Deliverer.*
You are our *Strength* and our *Peace.*
You are our *Joy* and our *Comfort.*
You are our *Salvation* and our *Guide.*
You are our *EVERYTHING.*

Lord, when things spin and twist and swirl, seemingly out of control, You are there keeping it all together. Praise be to You, and You alone.

By Your words I can see where I'm going;
they throw a beam of light on my dark path...
Everything's falling apart on me, GOD;
put me together again with Your Word.
Psalm 119:105 (THE MESSAGE)

Then Jesus again spoke to them, saying,
"I am the Light of the world; he who follows Me will not
walk in the darkness, but will have the Light of life."
John 8:12 (NASB)

A Note of HOPE
_____
_____
_____
_____
_____
_____
_____
_____
_____

In him we were also chosen...according to the plan of him who works out everything in conformity with the purpose of his will, in order that we...might be for the praise of his glory.
Ephesians 1:11-12

Why is truth so hard at times, Lord? This is one of those passages I find very difficult. Wonderful promises are contained here, but the hard and difficult are here as well.

I'm so grateful that I'm chosen by You, holy God. That truth is more marvelous than words could ever express. And You hand-picked _____, too. Amazing. All this perfect choosing is designed so that everything will conform to Your will, which we *know* is perfect.

But then I look at her cancer, and I wonder how it all fits together. How can this insidious disease *ever* be part and parcel of Your will? How, Lord? When I read further, I see where this is going. It's all for the praise of Your glory. Still, I have to shake my head at the *hardness* of it all.

God, I pray You will speak to _____'s heart and spirit about the daily opportunity to praise. Since the speaking of Your mighty name acknowledges Your glory, may that simple act be the strength she needs to continue putting one foot in front of the other on her journey.

I cry out to God Most High,
to God who will fulfill His purpose for me.
He will send help from heaven to rescue me,
disgracing those who hound me....
My God will send forth His unfailing love and faithfulness.
Psalm 57:2-3 (NLT)

Give thanks in all circumstances,
for this is God's will for you in Christ Jesus.
1 Thessalonians 5:18

A Note of HOPE

*Give me Your lantern and compass, give
me a map so I can find my way to the sacred
mountain, to the place of Your presence...Why
are you down in the dumps, dear Soul? Why are
you crying the blues? Fix my eyes on God—soon
I'll be praising again. He puts a smile on my
face. He's my God!*
Psalm 43:3, 5 (THE MESSAGE)

Dear Lord,

I still find myself in shock over this diagnosis. I know how determined this horrid disease is. If you're not touched by it in some way, you've dodged a deadly bullet. I just never really thought it would happen to us. I thought we'd be the lucky ones.

But now staggering truths knock us off center, as the *unthinkable* has become a part of our daily thoughts. O God, how we need Your grace and mercy. How we long for Your peace—a peace that infiltrates these *unthinkable thoughts* and wraps around them in restfulness. Tears flow. So does the fear.

Please light _____'s path and give her clear direction. Continue to draw her heart, soul, mind and spirit to You day-by-day, moment-by-moment. Let her find comfort in Your presence and envelop her in a peace she can't possibly understand.

As the tears fall, tenderly wipe them away with Your gentle hand.

There is a time for everything,
and a season for every activity under the heavens:
a time to be born and a time to die,
a time to plant and a time to uproot,
a time to kill and a time to heal,
a time to tear down and a time to build,
a time to weep and a time to laugh,
a time to mourn and a time to dance.
Ecclesiastes 3:1-4

I have told you these things, so that in Me you may have
(perfect) peace and confidence. In the world you have
tribulation and trials and distress and frustration; but be of
good cheer (take courage; be confident, certain, undaunted)!
For I have overcome the world. (I have deprived it of power
to harm you and have conquered it for you.)
John 16:33 (AMP)

A Note of HOPE

_____

_____

_____

_____

_____

_____

_____

But I am poor, sorrowful, and in pain; let Your salvation, O God, set me up on high.
*   I will praise the name of God with a song and will magnify Him with thanksgiving.*
Psalm 69:29-30 (AMP)

Lord,

We can all echo these words at one time or another. Despair hits. Fear reigns. Uncertainty looms. These feelings are normal and nothing to be ashamed of. In fact, I'm experiencing a bit of this right now. Wondering, *praying*, worrying, *praying*, releasing, *praying*, begging, *praying*, resting and *praying*. It all just keeps rolling around into one big circle of *prayer* for my dear _____.

Be with her today, Jesus, as she wonders and worries and releases and begs and rests and prays. It's perfectly understandable for her to go through *all* these feelings time and time and time again. Pain and distress are part of this journey, but it's so vital for her...for me...to move to the second part of this passage and not just "tread water" in the first five words.

Lord, in everything that _____ is experiencing right now, I ask You to urge her to praise Your name and glorify You with thanksgiving. Remind *both* of us that the thankfulness pleases You, that praise delights Your heart. How we need to remember this each and every day through each and every circumstance.

But when they in their trouble turned to the Lord,
the God of Israel, and [in desperation earnestly] sought Him,
He was found by them.
2 Chronicles 15:4 (AMP)

I've learned by now to be quite content whatever my
circumstances. I'm just as happy with little as with much,
with much as with little. I've found the recipe for being
happy whether full or hungry, hands full or hands empty.
Whatever I have, wherever I am, I can make it through
anything in the One who makes me who I am.
Philippians 4:11-13 (THE MESSAGE)

A Note of HOPE

_____

_____

_____

_____

_____

_____

_____

_____

_____

_____

What would have become of me had I not believed that I would see the Lord's goodness in the land of the living! Wait and hope for and expect the Lord; be brave and of good courage and let your heart be stout and enduring. Yes, wait for and hope for and expect the Lord.
Psalm 27:13-14 (AMP)

O Lord,

I remember well how I relied on this verse during my own cancer journey. I love that it says to wait, hope for and expect *You!* Not what You are going to *do*, but who You are going to *be!* That's a huge distinction. If my faith is based on what You do, then I'm going to be in for a wild ride. Your thoughts are not my thoughts, and Your ways are certainly not my ways; so if I think I'm going to be able to figure out *what* You are doing or *why* You are doing it, I had better think again!

Though the *what* and the *why* remain veiled...the *Who* never does. Everywhere we look, You are visible. Every blessing we receive is a gift from Your hand. We exist because You are mercy. We carry on because You are strength. We learn because You are patience. We rest assured because You are love.

May _____ be brave and of good courage as she waits, hopes for and expects *You!*

"For my thoughts are not your thoughts,
neither are your ways my ways,"
declares the Lord.
"As the heavens are higher than the earth,
so are my ways higher than your ways
and my thoughts than your thoughts."
Isaiah 55:8-9

The fundamental fact of existence is that this trust in God,
this faith, is the firm foundation under everything that
makes life worth living. It's our handle on what we can't see.
Hebrews 11:1 (THE MESSAGE)

A Note of HOPE

_____

_____

_____

_____

_____

_____

_____

_____

_____

_____

In the Heat of Battle

Prayers during Treatment

For I am convinced that neither death nor life, neither angels nor demons, neither the present nor the future, nor any powers, neither height nor depth, nor anything else in all creation, will be able to separate us from the love of God that is in Christ Jesus our Lord.
Romans 8:38-39

To the cancer patient

The battle. No one can fully prepare for this. Not really. There are so many pieces…physical breakdown, mental anguish, spiritual faltering. How can you be fully prepared for something you've never encountered before? Well-meaning and well-educated "others" can tell you what to expect, but the reactions and responses are yours, and yours alone.

To the Faithful Warrior
Let me urge you to pray. Don't let up!
Fighting is intense.
Ambushes are everywhere.
There is no rest on the front lines.

Rejoice and exult in hope; be steadfast and patient in suffering and tribulation; be constant in prayer.
Romans 12:12 (AMP)

Father God,

The diagnosis has revealed a need for more. We were hoping for a different answer, but it doesn't look like that's on the horizon. The surgery wasn't enough. Now further treatment is necessary. Chemotherapy. Radiation. It makes me sigh.

She was able to *"exult in hope"* when the cancer was found, knowing it could have gone much longer without being detected. But now she must step into that place of being *"patient in suffering and tribulation."* I sigh again.

Even if the treatment proves to be fairly smooth and easy for her, there is still the waiting and wondering. Waiting and wondering. Will anyone else think about that on a daily basis? How I pray so! Please give her family tremendous sensitivity during this period of time. Let them ask, let them listen and let them enfold her with love and support.

Lord, give _____ the stamina, both physically and emotionally, to weather this approaching storm. I think these will be some of her darkest days, not much light sifting through the heavy clouds. But I also believe these can be some of her sweetest days as she discovers new ways to draw close to Your heart.

I'm grateful, Lord, so very grateful for all You're doing on her behalf.

Be still and rest in the Lord;
wait for Him and patiently lean yourself upon Him.
Psalm 37:7 (AMP)

Be assured that from the first day we heard of you, we
haven't stopped praying for you, asking God to give you wise
minds and spirits attuned to His will, and so acquire a
thorough understanding of the ways in which God works...
We pray that you'll have the strength to stick it out over the
long haul—not the grim strength of gritting your teeth but
the glory-strength God gives. It is strength that endures the
unendurable and spills over into joy, thanking the Father
who makes us strong enough to take part in everything
bright and beautiful that He has for us.
Colossians 1:9, 11, 12 (THE MESSAGE)

A Note of HOPE

_____

_____

_____

_____

_____

_____

_____

_____

_____

_____

*We demolish arguments and every pretension
that sets itself up against the knowledge of God,
and we take captive every thought to make it
obedient to Christ.*
    2 Corinthians 10:5

Lord,

Please put a hedge of protection around _____'s thoughts. Keep her safe from the fiery darts of the enemy. He's so skilled at firing off arrows of fear, worry and dread when we least expect it. Oh, how he loves to catch us unprepared! Instead, Lord, may he run into a resilient shield of holy protection. A shield held in place by Your very words of confidence, peace and steadiness. A shield held in place by _____'s ever-trusting, ever-worshiping hands. Though the enemy comes to steal her peace, kill her joy and destroy her hope, I ask You to protect and defend Your precious child.

Fill her thoughts with powerful, encouraging Scripture. Let her meditate on *what is* and not *what if!* "*Whatever is true, whatever is noble, whatever is right, whatever is pure, whatever is lovely, whatever is admirable*" (Philippians 4:8). Let the *what is* of this verse permeate and dispel all the *what ifs* in her heart, soul, mind and spirit. Strengthen her to make good thought choices. If there is anything excellent or praiseworthy about her situation may her thoughts find their home there.

We wait in hope for the Lord;
he is our help and our shield.
In him our hearts rejoice,
for we trust in his holy name.
May your unfailing love be with us, Lord,
even as we put our hope in you.
Psalm 33:20-22

The thief comes only in order to steal and kill and destroy.
I came that they may have and enjoy life and have it in
abundance (to the full, till it overflows).
John 10:10 (AMP)

A note of HOPE

_____

_____

_____

_____

_____

_____

_____

_____

_____

_____

And so, Lord, where do I put my hope? My only
hope is in You.
Psalm 39:7 (NLT)

Yes, Lord, I'm hoping. Always hoping. Treatment has just begun for _____ and what lies ahead is yet to be seen. We live in a fallen world filled with sin and disease, but still You remain in control…still You remain faithful. Thank You for that solid truth on which we can confidently place our hope.

In the midst of every uncertainty and every question she faces, let *hope* and *faith* be the "bookends" holding everything upright in her life. She will go through a multitude of emotions, but I ask You to keep her steady all the way through them, never letting her get too discouraged before *hope* and *faith* prop her back up again.

How I pray she will wake up each morning with *hope* in her heart and lay her head on the pillow at night with a growing *faith* within her soul. With those strong "bookends" in place, I have to believe she will be just fine.

*But joyful are those who have
the God of Israel as their helper,
whose hope is in the Lord their God.
He made heaven and earth,
the sea, and everything in them.
He keeps every promise forever.*
Psalm 146:5-6 (NLT)

*Now faith is confidence in what we hope for
and assurance about what we do not see.*
Hebrews 11:1

A Note of HOPE

_____

_____

_____

_____

_____

_____

_____

_____

_____

_____

And this is my prayer: that your love would abound more and more in knowledge and depth of insight.
Philippians 1:9

Be with _____ today. Send her news this morning of Your unfailing love. As she reads Your Word or turns her heart to prayer, let an overwhelming sense of Your incredible, infinite love wash over her.

A Love that compels You to stay with her, whether she rises to the heights or sinks to the depths.

A Love that compels You to think about her more times than she could possibly count.

A Love that compels You to pour grace-filled compassion on her life.

A Love that compels You to give only good and perfect gifts.

A Love that compels You to do exceedingly abundantly beyond her imagination.

A Love that compels You to rejoice over her with heavenly singing.

Because of this Love, may she have a spring in her step, a song in her heart and a smile on her lips. May the love You show _____ be reflected in the love she shows others.

*The Lord is my Strength and my [impenetrable] Shield;
my heart trusts in, relies on, and confidently leans on Him,
and I am helped; therefore my heart greatly rejoices,
and with my song will I praise Him.*
Psalm 28:7 (AMP)

*But he said to me, "My grace is sufficient for you,
for my power is made perfect in weakness."
Therefore I will boast all the more gladly about my
weaknesses, so that Christ's power may rest on me.*
2 Corinthians 12:9

A Note of HOPE

> *Whom have I in heaven but you? And earth has nothing I desire besides you. My flesh and my heart may fail, but God is the strength of my heart and my portion forever.*
> **Psalm 73:25, 26**

Let me breathe this in as I pray for_____. Flood her heart, soul, mind and spirit with this empowering, freeing truth. It's You, Lord! It's always You! The trappings of earth really hold nothing for us, for our life is hidden with You in the heavenly places.

Father, _____'s "flesh" appears to be failing; yet You hold her in Your mighty hand. Don't let her "heart" fail in the midst of this struggle, though discouragement presses in hard. Be her Strength, her Hope, her Joy, her Promise, her Helper, her Deliverer, her EVERYTHING.

May she come to know the sweetest, most intimate fellowship with You as You draw close to her on a daily basis. Teach her new and wonderful things from Your Word. Comfort her with Your tenderness.

Sing a new song with _____ today. A song of Your love and faithfulness, followed tomorrow by a song of Your grace and truth. Just keep adding new verses, Lord, for they will never run out! Thank You for being our portion. An ample supply for all that we need.

He will cover you with his feathers,
and under his wings you will find refuge;
his faithfulness will be your shield and rampart.
Psalm 91:4

I have strength for all things in Christ Who empowers me
[I am ready for anything and equal to anything
through Him Who infuses inner strength into me;
I am self-sufficient in Christ's sufficiency].
Philippians 4:13 (AMP)

A Note of HOPE

---

*"Welcome, welcome, welcome. I welcome everything that comes to me today because I know it's for my healing."**

Everything? That's hard, God, but I think that's what You always ask of us. It's what propels us forward; it's what changes our perspective; it's what conforms us into the image of Your blessed Son. May _____ open her arms wide to accept *all* things... everything...throughout her journey. In her fear she might want to shrink back, afraid of the outcome, but I pray You would encourage her to "lean into" *all* that is placed before her. Lifted arms open wide and hands outstretched to whatever lies ahead.

*"I welcome all thoughts, feelings, emotions, persons, situations and conditions."**

Oh, to look at each and every day through this lens. So often we endure, accept and tolerate all thoughts, feelings, emotions, situations and conditions...but welcome them? Hardly!

Lord, please guide _____'s heart to welcome and embrace *all* that comes her way. As each phase of her treatment and recovery unfolds, may she welcome *all* that it holds, knowing You are working everything for good and for her ultimate healing. "Welcome, welcome, welcome"! May that be her brave new song.

In their peril their courage melted away....
Then they cried out to the Lord in their trouble,
and he brought them out of their distress.
Psalm 107:26, 28

Consider it a sheer gift, friends, when tests and challenges
come at you from all sides. You know that under pressure,
your faith-life is forced into the open and shows
its true colors. So don't try to get out of anything
prematurely. Let it do its work so you become mature
and well-developed, not deficient in any way.
James 1:2-4 (THE MESSAGE)

*The Welcoming Prayer by Father Thomas Keating

A Note of HOPE

_____

_____

_____

_____

_____

_____

_____

_____

_____

_____

*"I let go of my desire for power and control."**

Power and control. How we fight for them. From our first breath to our last, we grasp for that which is never going to be ours. Lord, You tell us to relinquish them, to quit struggling, but still we struggle on.

I think the word "desire" is the key. Please help _____ to place herself fully and peacefully in Your safe, loving hands. Let her rest in the confidence that You are for her, You will never leave her, Your plans for her include a future and a hope.

*"I let go of my desire for survival and security."**

This next phrase is more-than-likely a deal-breaker for most people. Survival and security. How can we possibly let go of our desire for those? Survival and security are a basic fiber of who we are as people. Lord, how could we possibly step away from that inward, driving need? Maybe it goes back to the word "desire" again? It all feels like layers, Lord, having to peel them off one by one to get to the most important, vital, vibrant center of it all. Please help her to strengthen her moment-by-moment, situation-by-situation trust in You. It's the blessed, heart-depth realization that our home...our true place of residence...is with You.

*He who dwells in the shelter of the Most High will rest in
the shadow of the Almighty. I will say of the Lord,
"He is my refuge and my fortress, my God, in whom I trust."*
Psalm 91:1-2

*And set your minds and keep them set on what is above
(the higher things), not on the things that are on the earth.*
Colossians 3:2 (AMP)

*The Welcoming Prayer by Father Thomas Keating

A Note of HOPE

_____

_____

_____

_____

_____

_____

_____

_____

_____

_____

"I let go of my desire to change any situation, condition, person or myself."*

Help _____ to be a woman who has learned to be content no matter what! Help her face every big and little thing with grace, patience and total trust in Your sovereign control of her life.

God, I ask You to give her a steady heart as she gets ready for her next step. After chemo, there will still be more to come. Surgery, more decisions, radiation, more decisions, and then more questions as to what else lies in front of her! A steady heart is an absolute must.

"I open to the love and presence of God and God's action within. Amen."*

Open. Ready. Vulnerable. Trusting. Willing. I pray that each one of these words would characterize _____'s entire being. May gates and doors fling open; may walls and barriers come crashing down. Fill _____in such a way that she's able to *welcome* Your perfect work in her life. O Lord, how I wish she didn't have to go through this, but it seems the way of suffering and sorrow is where You're leading her. She's traveled so far on this path of faith and determination, but she needs You to walk right beside her and to manifest Yourself in ways she can see and feel. It's only by Your grace that she continues to put one foot in front of the other.

When the trumpets sounded, the people shouted,
and at the sound of the trumpet, when the people gave
a loud shout, the wall collapsed.
Joshua 6:20

I have learned the secret of being content in any
and every situation, whether well fed or hungry,
whether living in plenty or in want. I can do all this
through him who gives me strength.
Philippians 4:12-13

*The Welcoming Prayer by Father Thomas Keating

A Note of HOPE

_____

_____

_____

_____

_____

_____

_____

_____

_____

_____

Be still and know (recognize and understand)
that I am God. I will be exalted among the
nations! I will be exalted in the earth!
Psalm 46:10 (AMP)

Dear God,

Please bless _____ today. Let her begin the blessed discovery of *be still and know that I am God* and let *me* continue on that journey of discovery with her.

Father, I ask You to ready her body for the next onslaught of chemo. So rough and aggressive. Please protect that which is healthy, targeting only that which is deadly to her. Give her strength and peace and contentment in the hard reality of the infusion room. I'm not sure how you learn contentment in that place, but I pray it would be so.

Keep her thoughts centered on You as she prepares to receive treatment. Enable her to focus on Your goodness and grace even in the midst of all that feels horrible and devastating. I know You're there with her...*for* her. God, please show Yourself in a very precious and powerful way today, allowing her to recognize You through the tears.

May You blanket her in Your love and warmth as she goes through this day. Walk with her, talk with her and assure her of Your abiding presence.

You rule the raging of the sea;
when its waves arise, You still them.
Psalm 89:9 (AMP)

A furious squall came up, and the waves broke over the
boat, so that it was nearly swamped. Jesus was in the stern,
sleeping on a cushion. The disciples woke him and said to
him, "Teacher, don't you care if we drown?" He got up,
rebuked the wind and said to the waves, "Quiet! Be still!"
Then the wind died down, and it was completely calm.
Mark 4:37-39

A Note of HOPE

He shouts with joy because you give him victory.
For you have given him his heart's desire; You
have withheld nothing he requested.
Psalm 21:1-2 (NLT)

Dear Lord,

What do You have in store for _____ today? What blessings are ready for delivery? Already You have blessed her with air in her lungs, life-blood flowing through her veins and a mind that is clear and quick. But wait…there's more! New mercies, unmerited favor, everlasting kindness, unconditional love, the mind of Christ, the indwelling Holy Spirit, full and open access to the throne of grace and personal communication with You, the Almighty God, the Great I AM, the Alpha and Omega.

Even with *so much*, I come to You asking for *more*. I ask You to give her the dreams and desires of her heart, blessing her with joy, contentment and healing. What a day it will be, God, when we can throw confetti and shout for joy over the victory You have given. Please continue to give patience, strength and hope to her and her family as they wait for that blessed day.

Dear Maker of heaven and earth, watch over _____ today. Don't let her foot slip, keep her from harm, and watch over her coming and going both today and forevermore!

Praise the Lord, my soul;
all my inmost being, praise his holy name.
Praise the Lord, my soul,
and forget not all his benefits—
who forgives all your sins
and heals all your diseases,
who redeems your life from the pit
and crowns you with love and compassion,
who satisfies your desires with good things
so that your youth is renewed like the eagle's.
Psalm 103:1-5

Let us then fearlessly and confidently and boldly draw near
to the throne of grace (the throne of God's unmerited favor to
us sinners), that we may receive mercy [for our failures] and
find grace to help in good time for every need [appropriate
help and well-timed help, coming just when we need it].
Hebrews 4:16 (AMP)

A Note of HOPE

_____

_____

_____

_____

_____

_____

Pushed to the wall, I called to God; from the wide open spaces He answered...I was right on the cliff edge, ready to fall, when God grabbed and held me. God's my strength, He's also my song; and now He's become my salvation.
Psalm 118:5, 13, 14 (THE MESSAGE)

O Lord,

I read these powerful, heartfelt words of the psalmist David and ask that they become _____'s words. May she call out to You, expecting an answer. May she sense Your grip on her life as the cliff edge looms ever closer, frightening and fierce. Be her song...her strength...her salvation.

I pray Your thorough, complete and absolute healing for _____. Is it too much to ask, Lord? I don't think so. I will ask it every day, a thousand times a day, if that's what it takes. Help me to stand *fully in faith*. Don't let me waver in my belief that *You are able* in this fight.

How I beg You to take her through this "valley of the shadow of death" with no spreading of this disease and no recurrence. Let there be only health in her future until the day You've planned to call her home to You.

Guard her heart and mind from fear and anxiety. Spread your perfect peace over her like a soothing balm. Make this all go away, Lord. Please!

O Lord my God, I called to you for help and you healed me.
O Lord, you brought me up from the grave;
you spared me from going down into the pit.
Psalm 30:2-3

So I say to you, "Ask and it will be given to you;
seek and you will find; knock and the door will be opened to
you. For everyone who asks receives; he who seeks finds;
and to him who knocks the door will be opened."
Luke 11:9-10

A Note of HOPE

_____

_____

_____

_____

_____

_____

_____

_____

_____

Surely you place them on slippery ground; you cast them down to ruin. How suddenly are they destroyed, completely swept away by terrors!
Psalm 73:18-19

I know you're talking about people here, Lord, but an enemy is an enemy! Place all that is cancerous and unhealthy on slippery ground. Take every errant cell, tissue and fiber and cast it down to complete and utter ruin…a holy "Take that!" Destroy them completely and sweep them away by Your power and might and perfect will.

This all makes me think of a heavenly video game, blasting intruders and obliterating the opposition. The internal fight that's going on in _____'s body is fierce, exhausting and discouraging. Please step right into the muddy middle of it all with Your overcoming, overwhelming strength.

"Do not be afraid or discouraged because of this vast army. For the battle is not yours, but God's" (2 Chronicles 29:15). I don't want to look at the vastness of this cancer army; I want to look only at *You* commanding this battle.

May _____stand strong in *faith*, cling tenaciously to *hope* and steep herself in Your abiding *love*. Is there any better battle plan than this, Lord?

Fear nothing—not wild wolves in the night,
not flying arrows in the day, not disease that prowls through
the darkness, not disaster that erupts at high noon.
Even though others succumb all around, drop like flies
right and left, no harm will even graze you.
Psalm 91:5-7 (THE MESSAGE)

Now these three remain: faith, hope and love.
But the greatest of these is love.
1 Corinthians 13:13

A Note of HOPE

_____

_____

_____

_____

_____

_____

_____

_____

_____

> *In this (new birth, living hope, unperishable inheritance, shielded by God's power, glorification) you greatly rejoice, though now for a little while you may have had to suffer grief in all kinds of trials. These have come so that your faith—of greater worth than gold, which perishes even though refined by fire—may be proved genuine and may result in praise, glory and honor when Jesus Christ is revealed.*
>
> *1 Peter 1:6-7 (emphasis mine)*

Father God,

May _____ continue to rejoice deep within her heart and spirit. May she keep herself centered on the *living hope*. So often the grief and sadness we feel because of our trials can completely overshadow the magnificent truths of these verses.

Father, help us, strengthen us, empower us to greatly rejoice while going through the refining process. Refining is hard. It hurts. It sometimes feels unfair. It can be lonely. But You have promised never to leave us or forsake us, and it is because of this truth we can hold onto *hope*.

Lord, I'm not sure whom I'm praying this for… myself or _____. You know both of our needs, weaknesses, desires and dreams, so I'm asking You to let Your grace and mercy rain down on each of our lives today.

*Praise be to the God and Father of our Lord Jesus Christ! In
his great mercy he has given us new birth into a living hope
through the resurrection of Jesus Christ from the dead, and
into an inheritance that can never perish, spoil or fade. This
inheritance is kept in heaven for you, who through faith are
shielded by God's power until the coming of the salvation
that is ready to be revealed in the last time.*
1 Peter 1:3-5

*I will bring that group through the fire
and make them pure.
I will refine them like silver
and purify them like gold.
They will call on My name,
and I will answer them.
I will say, "These are my people,"
and they will say, "The LORD is our God."*
Zechariah 13:9 (NLT)

A Note of HOPE

_____
_____
_____
_____
_____
_____
_____

I am still confident of this: I will see the goodness of the Lord in the land of the living. Wait for the Lord; be strong and take heart and wait for the Lord.

Psalm 27:13-14

Lord,

You are so good to us. Even when things are hard or sad or hurtful or confusing, You are still (and always) so good to us.

I await Your next round of goodness as You take _____ through radiation. That will be exhausting, for sure, but it will be one step closer to finishing her treatment. Give her family understanding when she needs to rest. Daily trips to the oncologist are going to be tiring, emotionally and physically.

I pray now for the technicians and staff who will be working with her. Give them tremendous compassion and skill. Take what is deadly (radiation) and transform it, by Your pure power, into something life-giving and beneficial.

Seek out any wandering cells and obliterate them. More combat to be done, Lord.

Most important in all this, I ask You to continue to build _____ in her faith and knowledge. Please give me opportunities to tell her of my prayers and to encourage her heart. How I pray she will dive deep into the wealth of who You are!

Yes, though I walk through the [deep, sunless] valley of the shadow of death, I will fear or dread no evil, for You are with me; Your rod [to protect] and Your staff [to guide], they comfort me. You prepare a table before me in the presence of my enemies. You anoint my head with oil; my [brimming] cup runs over. Surely or only goodness, mercy, and unfailing love shall follow me all the days of my life, and through the length of my days the house of the Lord [and His presence] shall be my dwelling place.
Psalm 23:4-6 (AMP)

"I am the Good Shepherd. The Good Shepherd lays down his life for the sheep…I am the Good Shepherd; I know my sheep and my sheep know Me."
John 10:11, 14

A Note of HOPE

The Lord is my shepherd,
I shall not want.
He makes me lie down in green pastures;
He leads me beside quiet waters.
He restores my soul;
He guides me in the paths of righteousness
For His name's sake....
Surely goodness and lovingkindness will follow me
All the days of my life,
And I will dwell in the house of the Lord forever.
Psalm 23:1-3, 6 (NASB)

This is one of those "breathe in, breathe out" passages of Scripture. It just brings a sense of calm peacefulness simply by reading it.

"The LORD is my Shepherd, I shall not be in want." Such precious words to my heart and soul. Be a gentle Shepherd for _____ today. Lead her to "green pastures" and "quiet waters" where she can find rest, nourishment and rejuvenation in Your presence. Let today be a blessed time of catching her breath. Inhale, exhale, and repeat.

Lord, with You as our Shepherd we have everything we need. Nothing is missing. Nothing is late. Nothing is wrong. Your constant care and provision for us are perfect.

In our daily lives be the gentle, quiet voice that speaks, the strong, steady hand that leads and the lavish fountain of grace that pours over our lives in magnificent abundance. "The Lord is my Shepherd, I shall not be in want."

I trust and pray that Your goodness and lovingkindness will follow _____ all the days of her life, and she will dwell in Your house forever.

*After the earthquake came a fire, but the Lord was not in
the fire. And after the fire came a gentle whisper.*
1 Kings 19:12

*And my God will liberally supply (fill to the full) your every
need according to His riches in glory in Christ Jesus.*
Philippians 4:19 (AMP)

A Note of HOPE

_____

_____

_____

_____

_____

_____

_____

_____

_____

_____

_____

> *But he said to me, "My grace is sufficient for you, for my power is made perfect in weakness." Therefore I will boast all the more gladly about my weaknesses, so that Christ's power may rest on me. That is why, for Christ's sake, I delight in weaknesses, in insults, in hardships, in persecutions, in difficulties. For when I am weak, then I am strong.*
> *2 Corinthians 12:9-10*

God. All grace. All goodness. All the time. (Breathe.)

In the peacefulness; in the noise and frenzy. In the overwhelming joy; in the heartbreaking sorrow. In the questions; in the answers. God. All grace. All goodness. All the time. (Breathe.)

Lord, our lives get so frenzied, so heartbroken, so overrun with questions. This swirling turmoil called *life* surrounds us, and we just need a moment to catch our spiritual and physical breath.

Father, I ask You to give _____ a day of blessed slowness. May she have the time to simply live in the moment as she gazes upon Your grace and Your goodness. Life swirls, but You stay steady. Life bucks, but You hold the reins. Life blurs, but You bring focus. O Lord, don't let her waste a single moment of Your all-the-time presence in her swirling, bucking, blurry phase of life.

For the Lord is good and his love endures forever;
his faithfulness continues through all generations.
Psalm 100:5

We don't yet see things clearly. We're squinting in a fog,
peering through a mist. But it won't be long before the
weather clears and the sun shines bright! We'll see it all then,
see it all as clearly as God sees us,
knowing Him directly just as He knows us!
1 Corinthians 13:12 (THE MESSAGE)

A Note of HOPE

_____

_____

_____

_____

_____

_____

_____

_____

_____

God...does great things which we cannot comprehend.
Job 37:5

Dear God,

The days continue to march along, one after the other. _____ is in the process of radiation and further cleansing of the cancer. I trust You to continue the work of perfect healing in her body, knowing that somehow, in some way, this is part of Your perfect plan.

Father, I ask that Your merciful, protective hand would be on her for the remainder of the radiation schedule. Too much pain with too many side effects, and here I thought this phase of treatment would be a walk in the park compared to chemo. I was wrong.

Be gracious to her, Lord. Please heal the places that are being burned and irritated because of this regimen. Spread a heavenly "numbing agent" over those rough, raw places, enabling her to function a bit more comfortably.

You are a *specific* God, so I *specifically* ask for this pinpoint, laser-accurate help and healing. Do the things we cannot comprehend, God. Do the things that are completely out of our human capability. Stay close to _____. Keep nudging her, hugging her, whispering to her, loving her and simply sharing the day with her. I don't know how anyone could walk this journey without You. It would be so lonely, Lord...so very lonely.

You are my lamp, O Lord; the Lord turns
my darkness into light. With your help I can advance against
a troop; with my God I can scale a wall.
As for God, his way is perfect; the word of the Lord is
flawless. He is a shield for all who take refuge in him.
2 Samuel 22:29-31

Then Jesus again spoke to them, saying,
"I am the Light of the world; he who follows Me will not
walk in the darkness, but will have the Light of life."
John 8:12 (NASB)

A Note of HOPE

As the deer longs for streams of water, so I long for you, O God. I thirst for God, the living God... Why am I discouraged? Why is my heart so sad? I will put my hope in God! I will praise Him again— my Savior and my God!
Psalm 42:1, 2, 5, 6 (NLT)

O Lord,

It's all getting to be too much for _____. This long (still unknown) haul is weighing on her heavily. She's weary, discouraged, tired and a bit hopeless. I know You can speak to all these feelings by Your Spirit, so that is what I ask.

Give her a fresh start today to endure the most difficult part of this journey. Prompt her to come to You for comfort and peace and then to come back again for even *more* comfort and *more* peace!

It brings tears to my eyes as I pray for her. Wouldn't You love to be able to sit with her and wrap her up in Your loving arms, soothing her in the precious way a mother soothes a troubled child? What a beautiful picture that brings to mind.

You are a tender, loving Father. You are my Savior and my God. This is what keeps me breathing prayers for grace and peace... grace and peace...grace and peace.

*Blessed be the Lord, who bears our burdens and
carries us day by day, even the God who is our salvation!
Selah [pause, and calmly think of that]!*
Psalm 68:19 (AMP)

And let the peace that comes from Christ rule in your hearts.
Colossians 3:15 (NLT)

A Note of HOPE

It is because of the Lord's mercy and loving-kindness that we are not consumed, because His [tender] compassions fail not. They are new every morning; great and abundant is Your stability and faithfulness.
Lamentations 3:22-23 (AMP)

Thank You for the freshness of this morning. We started over with brand new mercies the moment we opened our eyes! How we need Your grace and mercy to carry us through each and every day.

Father, please continue to reach Your healing hand out to_____. Use her treatment to target the cancer cells while still preserving all that is healthy and strong in her body. Put a mighty barrier around the cancerous cells. Don't let them spread, God!

I ask You to guard her heart and emotions today. Keep her focused on You and Your awesome strength and power. Don't let the enemy pull her thoughts to a place of doubt and discouragement.

We know *for certain* that You are in control of our lives.

We know *for certain* that Your love is without measure or bounds.

We know *for certain* that if You are for us, no one and nothing can stand against us.

Please, God, move these truths from simply what we know, to what we believe in our heart-of-hearts.

Your eyes saw my unformed body;
all the days ordained for me were written in your book
before one of them came to be.
Psalm 139:16

What, then, shall we say in response to these things?
If God is for us, who can be against us?
Romans 8:31

A Note of HOPE

_____

_____

_____

_____

_____

_____

_____

_____

_____

May the God of hope fill you with all joy and peace as you trust in him, so that you will overflow with hope by the power of the Holy Spirit.

Romans 15:13

Overflowing with hope! Not just a little trickle or a spoonful or a half cup or even up to the brim...but *overflowing*.

Overflowing with hope! Spilling all over everything and everyone around us...unable to contain it...having so much more than we need!

And what will cause our hope to overflow? Our moment-by-moment, situation-by-situation trust.

Lord, enable _____ to trust in Your abounding love for her, Your unending mercy surrounding her, Your grace pouring over her, Your cleansing forgiveness toward her and Your gentle patience with her.

Her job is to trust. Your job is to fill. As we place our daily faith in You, the promise to fully supply us with *joy* (in the midst of it all) and *peace* (in spite of it all) becomes obvious in our lives. O Lord, I continue to place _____ in Your hands and ask for joy and peace and hope and healing for all the way-too-difficult things in her life.

Lean on, trust in, and be confident in the Lord
with all your heart and mind and do not rely on your own
insight or understanding. In all your ways know,
recognize, and acknowledge Him, and He will
direct and make straight and plain your paths.
Proverbs 3:5-6 (AMP)

"Do not let your heart be troubled;
believe in God, believe also in Me.
John 14:1 (NASB)

A Note of HOPE

_____

_____

_____

_____

_____

_____

_____

_____

_____

_____

May He grant you your heart's desire and fulfill all your counsel! We will sing for joy over your victory, and in the name of our God we will set up our banners.
Psalm 20:4-5 (NASB)

Confetti. That's what we need, Lord. Confetti...lots of it. Bright, fluttering fragments of our heartfelt hallelujahs!

Waiting and watching and hoping. Praying and praying and praying some more. That's what we've all been doing, Lord, as the months have passed and the fight has been fought. She's been brave, valiant and courageous, and I'm so very proud of her. Now we wait and watch and hope, still praying for all things clear and clean and healed.

God, You are a God of restoration. You are a God of rebuilding. You are a God of rebirth. You have graciously guarded _____ throughout this entire process, bringing things to light and dispelling the darkness of this disease. How I thank You for that unending measure of faithfulness and grace in her life.

Until the final scan I will continue to stand firmly in faith as I stuff my pockets with confetti. We're all looking forward to hearing the "all clear" and having a colorful, joyful celebration of praise.

Give us help for the hard task; human help is worthless.
In God we'll do our very best;
He'll flatten the opposition for good.
Psalm 60:11-12 (THE MESSAGE)

Rejoice with those who rejoice (sharing others' joy),
and weep with those who weep (sharing others' grief).
Romans 12:15 (AMP)

A Note of HOPE

_____

_____

_____

_____

_____

_____

_____

_____

_____

Marching Home

Prayers for Remission or Release

***But one thing I do: forgetting what is behind
and straining toward what is ahead, I press on
toward the goal to win the prize for which God
has called me heavenward in Christ Jesus.***
Philippians 3:13-14

To the cancer patient

Scarred. Limping. Exhausted. Wondering…

Will the battle begin to rage again? Home free or free
to go "home"? There are no answers to those questions, at
least not here on earth. And so the "pressing on" begins in
a new way. Gaining strength. More strength than you ever
thought you'd need for a journey you hoped you'd never
have to make.

To the Faithful Warrior

Be a steady support as the march home begins.
Walk at their pace.
Rest when necessary.
Hold tightly to them.
Your faithful, calming presence is the ribbon
that continues to tie it all together.

I will exalt you, O Lord, for you lifted me out of the depths...O Lord, my God, I called to you for help, and you healed me. O Lord, you brought me up from the grave; you spared me from going down into the pit...you turned my wailing into dancing; you removed my sackcloth and clothed me with joy, that my heart may sing to you and not be silent. O Lord, my God, I will give you thanks forever.
Psalm 30:1-3, 11-12

Gracious Lord,

I speak Your holy Word over _____today, *knowing* it is alive and active and filled with power. Accept these words from the depth of my grateful heart.

Treatment is complete. That in itself is a reason for thankfulness and praise.

It took its toll, Lord, but how I pray it did its work. She was able to bear up under it, having the strong belief that You were using it to *lift her* and *help her* and *heal her*. The effects of it are still coursing through her body, so I will still pray this on-going trilogy to further this fight and win this battle.

I believe Your Word is *truth*...to lift her.

I believe Your Word is *power*...to help her.

I believe Your Word is *hope*...to heal her.

He raises the poor from the dust
and lifts the needy from the ash heap.
Psalm 113:7

When Jesus had entered Capernaum, a centurion came to
him, asking for help. "Lord," he said, "my servant lies
at home paralyzed, suffering terribly." Jesus said to him,
"Shall I come and heal him?" The centurion replied,
"Lord, I do not deserve to have you come under my roof.
But just say the word, and my servant will be healed."
Matthew 8:5-8

A Note of HOPE

_____

_____

_____

_____

_____

_____

_____

_____

_____

"I find that the great thing in this world is not so much where we stand, as in what direction we are moving."
Oliver Wendell Holmes

Dear Jesus,

Please keep _____ moving in the right direction. May she forget what lies behind in this cancer journey and continue to keep her hands stretched out for whatever lies ahead.

You've gone behind her, and You go before her. You walk her path in preparation for her footsteps. Please help her to place her "feet" in the exact "footprints" You've left behind—like walking in sand or snow and matching her steps stride for stride with You. Isn't that what we all want, Lord? Matching Your steps…staying in tune with Your Spirit…having our hearts beat with Yours? I shout a resounding YES!

May Your holy and perfect Presence be with _____ today. Whatever the day holds, would You hold her close to Your heart as You continue Your healing work in every cell, every fiber, every tissue and nuance of her being. May she embrace, with thankfulness and strength, *all* that lies before her as she presses on toward the goal.

Forget the former things;
do not dwell on the past.
See, I am doing a new thing!
Now it springs up; do you not perceive it?
I am making a way in the wilderness
and streams in the wasteland.
Isaiah 43:18-19

I'm not saying that I have this all together, that I have it
made. But I am well on my way, reaching out for Christ,
who has so wondrously reached out for me. Friends,
don't get me wrong: By no means do I count myself
an expert in all of this, but I've got my eye on the goal,
where God is beckoning us onward—to Jesus.
I'm off and running, and I'm not turning back.
Philippians 3:12-14 (THE MESSAGE)

A Note of HOPE

*Grace and peace to you from God our Father
and the Lord Jesus Christ.*
2 Corinthians 1:2

Are there any sweeter words than these? Is there a simpler, yet more profound, blessing than this? Truly I believe everything we need and desire is wrapped up in this one beautiful sentence.

Father God, I pray Your grace and peace upon _____. Let her exhale her expectations and simply breathe easy under Your wings. Shelter her, protect her, nourish her, heal her.

I know she thinks she should be "doing better." Maybe she *is* and just doesn't know it yet! Lord, she really needs to cut herself some slack. After all the chemo and all the radiation and all the changes to her very existence, she needs time to simply rest and recuperate. Please make a breakthrough here. It seems we're always ready to cut *others* some slack, but we find it hard to apply that to *ourselves*. Just human nature, I guess.

Right now it's still a waiting game for her. Is she in remission? Did it work? Is there more ahead for her?

As I prayed at the beginning, let me pray at the end...may Your grace and peace be upon _____'s life today and tomorrow and all the days following.

*You will guard him and keep him in perfect and
constant peace whose mind (both its inclination and its
character) is stayed on You, because he commits himself to
You, leans on You, and hopes confidently in You.
Isaiah 26:3 (AMP)*

*Now may the Lord of peace himself
give you peace at all times and in every way.
The Lord be with all of you.
2 Thessalonians 3:16*

A Note of HOPE

_____

_____

_____

_____

_____

_____

_____

_____

_____

_____

But the Counselor, the Holy Spirit, whom the Father will send in my name, will teach you all things and will remind you of everything I have said to you.

John 14:26

Dear God,

Let Your Holy Spirit guide _____ today. Help her to listen and act in accordance with Your will. Your Spirit is the Giver of Truth. He is the Wonderful Counselor for each situation she faces. He is the Comforter You sent to minister in times of sadness and pain. Help her to rely on Him in a more tangible, steadfast way, knowing He will never lead her astray.

Please teach her the habits of praying constantly, giving thanks through all circumstances and rejoicing steadily in You. These habits are strong cords that draw her to You and keep her so very close. Blessed be the tie that binds!

By Your grace and Your tender love, I ask You to touch _____'s life in a personal and precious way today. Bring her a gentle awareness of Your abiding presence. May she sense You shoulder to shoulder, yet just around every corner; never leaving her side, yet always going before her to prepare her way.

Please answer her prayers swiftly. Please satisfy the deepest longing of her heart. Please set her life in a place of joy and contentment. Let all that is within her bless Your holy name.

His names will be:
Amazing Counselor,
Strong God,
Eternal Father,
Prince of Wholeness.
Isaiah 9:6 (THE MESSAGE)

And I will ask the Father, and He will give
you another Comforter (Counselor, Helper,
Intercessor, Advocate, Strengthener, and Standby),
that He may remain with you forever.
John 14:16 (AMP)

A Note of HOPE

_____

_____

_____

_____

_____

_____

_____

_____

_____

_____

Be joyful in hope, patient in affliction, faithful in prayer.

Romans 12:12

Dear Jesus,

This precious woman has lived "*joyful in hope,*" she has journeyed through the land of "*patient in affliction,*" and now we have the final act, "*faithful in prayer.*" I wonder, Lord, who is this for? Her or me?

Maybe this is the call for me to get my "second wind," not forsaking the fervency of my earlier prayers when things were more critical and crisis-laden. Maybe this is the call for me to be even *more* committed in my prayers for her.

When You were in the Garden of Gethsemane, You asked Your disciples to pray...but they couldn't. They became weary and fell asleep, leaving You all alone in that place of anxiety and pain. O Lord, don't let that happen to me! I want to stand steadfast and strong alongside _____ for the remainder of this ordeal. I want to continue to lift her before Your throne of grace, begging for a full and complete remission.

Look at all she's been through. How could my weariness even matter in the grand scheme of things? Strengthen me to persevere in prayer. Strengthen her to *never* forego the fight.

Have you not known? Have you not heard? The everlasting God, the Lord, the Creator of the ends of the earth, does not faint or grow weary; there is no searching of His understanding. He gives power to the faint and weary, and to him who has no might He increases strength [causing it to multiply and making it to abound].
Isaiah 40:28, 29 (AMP)

So let's not allow ourselves to get fatigued doing good. At the right time we will harvest a good crop if we don't give up, or quit.
Galatians 6:9 (THE MESSAGE)

A Note of HOPE

_____

_____

_____

_____

_____

_____

_____

_____

_____

This is the day the Lord has made; let us rejoice and be glad in it.
Psalm 118:24

Sovereign Lord,

Today You are Worthy and Faithful and Righteous. Today You are Kind and Merciful and Loving. Today You are Forgiving and Patient and Gracious. Today You are Compassionate and Glorious and Just. Today You are Wonderful and Marvelous and True. Today You are Wise and Pure and Comforting. Lord, help us to live for today and today alone. It will have enough challenges to deal with that it makes absolutely no sense to worry or stress about tomorrow.

And You know what, Lord? *Tomorrow* will be *today* again! You are one continuous loop of power and presence in our lives. Oh, that we would stamp that on our hearts and live according to that freeing truth. May _____ be abundantly aware of who You are today, holding fast to Your marvelous attributes. Equip her to live this day with a heart of rejoicing.

Today You are mine, and I am yours. Today You are the Potter, and I am the clay. Today You are the Vine, and I am the branch. Today You are the Shepherd, and I am Your lamb. How grateful I am that You are the same yesterday, forever and today!

*Give your entire attention to what God is doing right now,
and don't get worked up about what may or may not
happen tomorrow. God will help you deal with whatever
hard things come up when the time comes.*
Matthew 6:34 (THE MESSAGE)

Yet you, LORD, are our Father.
We are the clay, you are the potter;
we are all the work of your hand.
Isaiah 64:8

A Note of HOPE

_____

_____
_____
_____
_____
_____
_____
_____
_____

The Lord bless you and keep you; the Lord make his face shine upon you and be gracious to you; the Lord turn his face toward you and give you peace.
Numbers 6:24-26

Father God,

There is such beauty in your smile…such sweetness. *Your* smile puts a smile on *my* face. Thank You for turning toward _____ today with Your glorious, comforting countenance. Give her vision and perspective to see You every step of the way, whether she's feeling sure-footed and stable or slipping and sliding.

Help her to find the gift in everything—*everything*—even in the hard "no matter whats." Be her strength and her shield. Strength to put one foot in front of the other on this treacherous path and her shield from further devastating disease.

Be her cure, Jesus! Her total, complete, forever-remission cure! During the stressful times of *waiting* and *wondering*, I ask You to fill her heart with joy and thankfulness. During the anxious times of *worrying* and *wishing*, please give her a huge bouquet of hope. What a beautiful picture that paints.

May her words of gratitude and praise release the miracle from Your hand. The miracle of Your presence and Your healing. May it be so, dear Lord.

Yet I will rejoice in the Lord, I will be joyful in God my Savior. The Sovereign Lord is my strength; he makes my feet like the feet of a deer, he enables me to go on the heights.
Habakkuk 3:18-19

May the God of hope fill you with all joy and peace as you trust in him, so that you may overflow with hope by the power of the Holy Spirit.
Romans 15:13

A Note of HOPE

Cast all your anxiety on him because he cares for you.

1 Peter 5:7

Precious Lord,

Please minister to _____ today. Whisper Your secrets to her this morning. Cleanse her heart and clear her cluttered mind by the sanctifying truth of Your Word. Life can be so hard, so discouraging. I ask You to assure her deep within her soul that You are the One who will never abandon the design process in her life. You *will* complete the good work You started in her. That is Your promise.

She doesn't have to "gut it out" alone or even in her own strength, for You, O God, walk beside her to strengthen and uphold her with Your righteous right hand. You know everything she is feeling, and You have promised to bear her burdens.

You are her *light*—illuminating her path.

You are her *salvation*—saving her from all that is harmful.

You are her *stronghold*—holding tight to her, never leaving or forsaking her.

Because of these powerful truths we never need to be afraid of what lies ahead!

*Blessed be the Lord, Who bears our burdens
and carries us day by day, even the God Who is our
salvation! Selah [pause, and calmly think of that]!*
Psalm 68:19 (AMP)

*Are you tired? Worn out? Burned out on religion? Come to
Me. Get away with Me and you'll recover your life. I'll show
you how to take a real rest. Walk with Me and work with
Me—watch how I do it. Learn the unforced rhythms of
grace. I won't lay anything heavy or ill-fitting on you. Keep
company with Me and you'll learn to live freely and lightly.*
Matthew 11:28-29 (THE MESSAGE)

A Note of HOPE

All the days ordained for me were written in
your book before one of them came to be.
Psalm 139:16

Sovereign Lord,

Today I don't like this verse. I don't like it at all. I've talked about it, shared it, believed it, delighted in it and trusted it. But today I don't like it, and I don't want to think about what it really and truly means.

What if all the praying and hoping and trusting don't bring about the desired result? What if the days ordained for _____ are far less than what any of us would want? What do we do then, Lord? What do we do?

I hate this. I really do. I know that I need to pray, "Thy will be done," but I'm having a difficult time wrapping my head around that prayer. I want *my* will. I want her to stay here with us. I want her to make it through this with flying colors and perfect healing! But it can't be my will, can it, Lord? Though I don't understand it, I know *Your* will is the only perfect and right one. You are God. I am not.

Lord, I ask You to strengthen each person in this story. Enable us to be the people we need to be for _____. Teach us how to be *Your* hands and feet and voice—ours simply will not suffice.

*I know that You can do all things, and that no thought
or purpose of Yours can be restrained or thwarted.*
Job 42:2 (AMP)

*To him who is able to keep you from stumbling and to
present you before his glorious presence without fault and
with great joy—to the only God our Savior be glory, majesty,
power and authority, through Jesus Christ our Lord,
before all ages, now and forevermore! Amen.*
Jude 24-25

A Note of HOPE

The Lord confides in those who fear him; he makes his covenant known to them.
Psalm 25:14

Let me rewrite this one...

"Jesus whispers His secrets to His children as they live in loving, awe-filled submission to His lordship; He reveals His eternal promises to them."

O Lord, this is just so beautiful...so encouraging. To think that the Maker of heaven and earth would bend down to whisper in my ear is so very lovely! Lord, please draw close to _____ today. Speak words of kindness, hope and healing to her heart. Whisper sweet *everythings* to her, filling her with strength, endurance and patience.

May she live in submission to Your will in the "no matter what" and the "no matter when." No one knows how long she'll be traveling this road or what lies ahead on her journey, but we can be fully confident that You are already there with a huge storehouse of Your eternal promises. Promises that will meet her every need— promises as sure as the rising and setting of the sun.

Jesus, thank You for faithfully cheering her on every step of the way. Thank You for the beautiful "bouquet" of blessings You have waiting for her at the finish line. She's going to love it!

You hem me in behind and before,
and you lay your hand upon me.
Such knowledge is too wonderful for me,
too lofty for me to attain.
Where can I go from your Spirit?
Where can I flee from your presence?
If I go up to the heavens, you are there;
if I make my bed in the depths, you are there.
If I rise on the wings of the dawn,
if I settle on the far side of the sea,
even there your hand will guide me,
your right hand will hold me fast.
Psalm 139:5-10

And let us run with patient endurance and steady and active
persistence the appointed course of the race that is set before us.
Hebrews 12:1 (AMP)

A Note of HOPE

_____

_____

_____

_____

_____

"Standing on the promises I cannot fall,
Listening every moment to the Spirit's call,
Resting in my Savior as my all in all,
Standing on the promises of God."
Excerpt from "Standing on the Promises" in
Songs of Faith and Praise

Good morning, Lord.

The day is new, and so is Your mercy. Oh, how we need it. I wonder what You have up Your sleeve for today? I know there are blessings all lined up, ready to be delivered. I know Your faithfulness tank is full and functioning. I know Your grace is poised to write a new story of sufficiency.

All these things bring a smile to my face and a peace to my heart. Bottom line for every single day, every hour, every moment and every breath is this:

You've got it covered.

Plain, simple, true.

Shower my dear _____ with that knowledge. Speak to the innermost part of her being with the depth of this blessed assurance. She needs that today, Lord. In the midst of new questions and new fears and new frustrations, please settle her into the soft, cozy center of Your promises.

*It is because of the Lord's mercy and loving-kindness
that we are not consumed, because His [tender] compassions
fail not. They are new every morning; great and abundant
are Your stability and faithfulness. The Lord is my portion
or share, says my living being (my inner self); therefore
will I hope in Him and wait expectantly for Him.*
Lamentations 3:22-24 (AMP)

*By His divine power, God has given us everything we need
for living a godly life. We have received all of this by coming
to know Him, the one who called us to Himself by means of
His marvelous glory and excellence. And because of His glory
and excellence, He has given us great and precious promises.*
2 Peter 1:3-4 (NLT)

A Note of HOPE

_____

_____

_____

_____

_____

_____

_____

_____

_____

_____

At this, Job...fell to the ground in worship and said... "The Lord gave and the Lord has taken away; may the name of the Lord be praised." In all this, Job did not sin by charging God with wrongdoing.
Job 1:20-22

God,

I'm not as strong as Job. I'm just not. As I swallow back tears I'm having a really hard time not blaming You. I'm sorry, Lord. I know I shouldn't, but You're the only One who could have made this story end differently...but You didn't.

I just don't understand why You would let _____ die. Oh, I know You can still come in with a last-minute rescue, but somehow I don't see that coming. We've all prayed and prayed and prayed, but there are no indications of healing, miraculous or otherwise. Why, God? Why?

What's her family going to do without her, Lord? What am I going to do without her? This is too much to bear...too much to hold in my heart. I can't seem to find any more hope-filled words.

Now I'll simply pray for peace. Peace for her remaining days... peace for all those who love her. Oh, how did we *ever* get to this place? Only You can bring comfort far beyond anything *anyone* could possibly say. I just keep relying on that, Lord.

To all who mourn…He will give a crown of beauty for ashes,
a joyous blessing instead of mourning, festive praise
instead of despair. In their righteousness, they will be
like great oaks that LORD has planted for His own glory.
Isaiah 61:3 (NLT)

May God our Father and the Lord Jesus Christ
give you grace and peace. All praise to God, the Father
of our Lord Jesus Christ. God is our merciful Father
and the source of all comfort.
2 Corinthians 1:2, 3 (NLT)

A Note of HOPE

_____

_____

_____

_____

_____

_____

_____

_____

_____

_____

Meanwhile, the moment we get tired in the waiting, God's Spirit is right alongside helping us along. If we don't know how or what to pray, it doesn't matter, He does our praying in and for us, making prayer out of our wordless sighs, our aching groans.
Romans 8:26 (THE MESSAGE)

O Lord,

I truly am tongue-tied today. There are no words...no sentences...no semblance of intelligent articulation.

I need You. She needs You. That's about all I can say. Yet I know in the depth of my very soul that is the *most* I can say.

Let Your Spirit help each of us today. Weaknesses abound. Questions remain unanswered. Prayers don't seem to reach beyond the ceiling.

There are no words, Lord. None at all. But when there *are* no words, this I know without a doubt...You are there to fill up all the empty spaces and heal all the broken places.

Dear Jesus, please let Your Spirit intercede for _____ today. May He come before the Eternal Father with deep petitions unleashed from a place of perfect wisdom and unmeasured love.

I need You to take over where my feeble words fall so miserably short. All I can do today is cry.

Out of the depths I cry to you, O Lord; O Lord, hear my voice. Let your ears be attentive to my cry for mercy...I wait for the Lord, my soul waits, and in his word I put my hope.
Psalm 130:1, 2, 5

And He Who searches the hearts of men knows what is in the mind of the [Holy] Spirit [what His intent is], because the Spirit intercedes and pleads [before God] in behalf of the saints according to and in harmony with God's will.
Romans 8:27 (AMP)

A Note of HOPE

_____

_____

_____

_____

_____

_____

_____

_____

_____

_____

_____

Teach us to number our days, that we may gain a heart of wisdom.
Psalm 90:12

Dear Lord,

My heart is filled with thoughts about _____. My breathing in and breathing out turn into one long, deep sigh. That which was contained and treated is no longer staying behind its boundary. The dam has been breached. The disease has overflowed.

O God, I have prayed and prayed and prayed that Your perfect, thorough healing would be a part of this plan, but with this latest metastasis, it appears that's not going to happen.

Why, Lord? Why? How could it be a problem for You to leave her here with us? Would it be such a travesty to alter Your plan? Would the world tilt off its axis and get off kilter if she stayed on the planet for several more years?

I know, I know…my thoughts and ways will *never* be able to line up fully with Yours. I know. It just shatters my heart to think about it.

For today, may my sweet _____ think small, making *everything* important. Since she's not able to think big anymore, may she realize, in a very profound way, that there is *no* insignificant moment. Enable her to look at each and every day as a precious gift.

*Who has scooped up the ocean in His two hands or
measured the sky between His thumb and little finger,
who has put all the earth's dirt in one of His baskets,
weighed each mountain and hill? Who could ever
have told God what to do or taught him His business?
What expert would He have gone to for advice...?*
Isaiah 40:12-14 (THE MESSAGE)

*And we know that in all things God works
for the good of those who love him, who have
been called according to his purpose.*
Romans 8:28

A Note of HOPE

_____

_____

_____

_____

_____

_____

_____

_____

_____

_____

God is our Refuge and Strength [mighty and impenetrable to temptation], a very present and well-proved help in trouble. Therefore we will not fear, though the earth should change and though the mountains be shaken into the midst of the seas, though its waters roar and foam, though the mountains tremble at its swelling and tumult. Selah [pause, and calmly think of that]!

Psalm 46:1-3 (AMP)

Trouble. Fear. Change. Tumult. O Lord, these are the feelings that are cascading through our lives. These are the emotions that are pouring into every crack and crevice of our being. All that used to be stable is changing and shaking, roaring and foaming. It's not working, Lord! The treatment is not holding back this army of cancerous cells. It appears we're out of answers. So now what do we do?

We pray. But we also need to hunker down and draw from *everything* we know about You. Remind our spirits of all You've been and done in the past. Remind our hearts how to trust You fully even in the midst of such grave disappointment. Let us live and breathe *Selah*—pausing and thinking about Your magnificence, Your power, Your sovereign control, Your holiness, Your provision, Your kindness.

Give _____ an overwhelming sense of *Selah*. Let her find rest and comfort in Your presence. Let her find strength and assurance in Your Word. Let her find a quiet place simply to lay her head on Your shoulder and cry.

When the earth and all its people quake,
it is I who hold its pillars firm.
Psalm 75:3

Blessed are those who mourn, for they will be comforted.
Matthew 5:4

A Note of HOPE

_____

_____

_____

_____

_____

_____

_____

_____

_____

_____

Lord, if you are willing... .
Luke 5:12

Almighty God,

I bow in worship to Your sovereign power today. I know You can heal _____, but I also know Your *perfect will* determines whether or not that happens. For as long as I live I will grapple with the hardness of this truth.

Lord, today I'm drawn to the story of the paralytic. I need to look deeper into this picture of faith and commitment.

"When Jesus returned to Capernaum several days later, the news spread quickly that He was back home. Soon the house where He was staying was so packed with visitors that there was no more room, even outside the door. While He was preaching God's word to them, four men arrived carrying a paralyzed man on a mat. They couldn't bring him to Jesus because of the crowd, so they dug a hole through the roof above His head. Then they lowered the man on his mat, right down in front of Jesus" (Mark 2:1-12, NLT).

The paralytic's friends were concerned, determined, persistent, willing to work, united in purpose, filled with faith and expectant. Isn't that how *we* should be whenever we come to You in prayer?

I'm coming to You today feeling persistent, determined and expectant. I bring _____ to You, holding a *big faith* in my heart that You are finishing up Your full, complete, perfect healing in her body. Jesus, You saw the faith of the paralytic's friends and gave the *blessing* of healing; now I ask that You would see mine, too! Lord, if there's any room in Your will for this blessing in her life, I pray it would be so.

Since a man's days are already determined,
and the number of his months is wholly in Your control...
he cannot pass the bounds of his allotted time.
Job 14:5 (AMP)

The earnest (heartfelt, continued) prayer
of a righteous man makes tremendous power
available (dynamic in its working).
James 5:16 (AMP)

A Note of HOPE

_____

_____

_____

_____

_____

_____

_____

_____

_____

I call on you, O God, for you will answer me;
give ear to me and hear my prayer. Show me the
wonder of your great love, you who save by your
right hand those who take refuge in you from
their foes. Keep me as the apple of your eye; hide
me in the shadow of your wings.
Psalm 17:6-8

We call. You answer. We talk. You listen. We take refuge. You show us the safety of Your great love. We are the apple of Your eye, and You spread Your protection over us. Amazing!

My heart is encouraged when I read that You save "those who take refuge in You." Thank You, Lord, for that reminder. You didn't say those who perform beautifully or never make mistakes. You didn't mention those who have a nonstop faith or serve happily in ministry. You didn't even talk about those who can quote pages of Bible verses or do missionary work overseas. What You did say is…

You are there for Your children who run to You for help!

_____ still needs Your help, Lord. She's not out of the woods, by any means. I ask You to keep the cancer in check while You build and fortify all that is healthy within her. Oh, we wait for the blessed day when this is only a distant memory.

In the meantime, please give _____ peace and assurance of Your constant hand on her life. Let her walk in confidence, not in fear.

GOD told them, "I've never quit loving you and never will.
Expect love, love, and more love!
And so now I'll start over with you
and build you up again...
You'll resume your singing,
grabbing tambourines and joining the dance."
Jeremiah 31:3, 4 (THE MESSAGE)

For God did not give us a spirit of timidity (of cowardice,
of craven and cringing and fawning fear), but
[He has given us a spirit] of power and of love and of calm
and well-balanced mind and discipline and self-control.
2 Timothy 1:7 (AMP)

A Note of HOPE

_____

_____

_____

_____

_____

_____

_____

_____

_____

_____

The name of the Lord is a strong tower; the righteous run to it and are safe.
Proverbs 18:10

Your name is Glorious.
Your name is Magnificent.
Your name is Power.
Your name is Protection.
Your name is Secure.
Your name is Strength.
Your name is Healing.
Your name is Abundance.
Your name is Faithful.
Your name is Love.

Dear Lord,

YOUR NAME is our strong and mighty tower. A place to run when we are frightened or under attack. I love that Your Word says, "Your name," and nothing more. I think there are many times in our lives when all we can do is whisper Your name. But in that whispering, wonderful blessings and attributes from heaven are released. Thank You, Lord.

May _____ speak out Your glorious, magnificent, powerful, protecting, secure, strengthening, healing, abundant, faithful, loving name today. Whether it is a joyous shout from the rooftop or a fragile whisper from a darkened room, please unleash *all* of who You are into her life.

Those who know your name trust in you,
for you, Lord, have never forsaken those who seek you.
Psalm 9:10

Therefore God exalted him to the highest place
and gave him the name that is above every name,
that at the name of Jesus every knee should bow,
in heaven and on earth and under the earth,
and every tongue acknowledge that Jesus Christ is Lord,
to the glory of God the Father.
Philippians 2:9-11

A Note of HOPE

*He calmed the storm to a whisper and stilled the
waves. What a blessing was that stillness as He
brought them safely into harbor!*
Psalm 107:29-30 (NLT)

A safe harbor. A place of rest. A shelter from the storm. Each
of these pictures brings a sense of peace and a wonderful feeling
of calm. After everything _____'s been through, this complete
sense of serenity is so very welcome, so very needed.

Lord, You've walked with her the entire way. You've been her
peace over the many months and "miles" of this arduous journey.
Oh, the idea of actually getting to this tranquil place, of being able
to breathe easy, seems almost too good to be true.

Is she past the worst of it now? Is it okay to settle back into a
normal routine without always looking over her shoulder? I can't
tell You what a blessed relief that would be, Lord.

You have been so faithful to _____. I know there were times
when she felt alone, forsaken, but You never left her side for a
moment. You couldn't. Your "heartstrings" *always* keep You close
to her with Your love and grace and mercy.

Oh, the sweet mercies of this cancer. I never thought I could
thank You for this, but I do. I thank You for the tenderness You've
shown and the faith You've nurtured in her life. It's been such a
blessing to have been a part of it all.

My gratitude overflows, dear Lord…so do my tears.

*You will guard him and keep him in perfect and
constant peace whose mind [both its inclination and its
character] is stayed on You, because he commits himself
to You, leans on You, and hopes confidently in You.
Isaiah 26:3 (AMP)*

*So humble yourselves under the mighty power of God,
and at the right time He will lift you up in honor. Give all
your worries and cares to God, for He cares about you.
1 Peter 5:6-7 (NLT)*

A Note of HOPE

_____

_____

_____

_____

_____

_____

_____

_____

_____

You did it: You changed wild lament into whirling dance; You ripped off my black mourning band and decked me with wildflowers. I'm about to burst with song; I can't keep quiet about You. God, my God, I can't thank You enough.
Psalm 30:11-12 (THE MESSAGE)

Thank you, Lord! Thank you!

Chemotherapy? Check. Radiation? Check. Cancer free? Check!

Lord, there are no words for what I'm feeling right now. How I praise You for doing the miraculous and marvelous in _____'s life. You are indeed a great and awesome God.

She's so relieved. We all are. I think I've been holding my breath for months now as she went through the exhausting, difficult treatment. Oh, how I wish there had been an easier path to take, but how I thank You for bringing her to this place of healing and health.

Now I ask that You would continue to build all that is strong and vital within her, constructing a road block to anything harmful or unhealthy. May her days be long and prosperous and filled with blessings from Your hand.

O Lord, I just want to go out and spin and shout and dance for joy! You did it, Lord! You did it!

I will exalt you, my God and King,
and praise your name forever and ever.
I will praise you every day;
yes, I will praise you forever.
Great is LORD! He is most worthy of praise!
No one can measure his greatness.
Let each generation tell its children of your mighty acts;
let them proclaim your power.
I will meditate on your majestic, glorious splendor
and your wonderful miracles.
Your awe-inspiring deeds will be on every tongue;
I will proclaim your greatness.
Everyone will share the story of your wonderful goodness;
they will sing with joy about your righteousness.
Psalm 145:1-7

A Note of HOPE

_____

_____

_____

_____

_____

_____

_____

_____

_____

_____

Afterword

If you've made it to this page then you've made a journey of prayer for someone who is very important to your heart. I know it was hard for you, but I applaud how you pushed your way through the pain to pray and pray and pray.

The road was rough, but I hope you encountered blessings and grace along the way. I also hope that your faith grew as you sensed God's presence over the weeks and months. Maybe you wrote some personal "HOPE notes" along the way; maybe you couldn't. Either way, let me encourage you to pass this book to the precious woman you've been praying for. I guarantee it will be an expression of love and encouragement to her. She will be blessed.

Now as we part company, dear reader, let me say this: Thank you for your partnership in the gospel. Thank you for praying without ceasing. Thank you for fighting the good fight.

Grace and peace to you, Faithful Warrior,

Katherine

About the Author

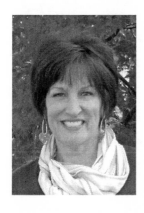

Katherine Hedlund, cancer survivor since 2000, fully understands the emotions, fears and questions facing the cancer sufferer. *Faithful Warrior* is a result of her commitment to prayer journaling intertwined with her love for God's Word. Katherine's writing is honest, encouraging and laced with tears. She knows what it is like to fight for her own personal healing as well as begging God's mercy and grace for others battling this terrible disease.

In addition to authoring *Faithful Warrior*, she writes a weekly blog at www.faithfulwarriorbook.com and www.FoundationForFamilies.org, providing an opportunity to teach and inspire her readers as she approaches God's Word in a practical, prayerful way.

Born and raised in Southern California, Katherine now resides in Rochester Hills, Michigan, with her husband, Gary, her "just-around-the-corner" adult children, Eric, Holly and Bryce, and her first Love-Love, grandson Austin.

Resources

Fettke, Tom. *The Hymnal for Worship and Celebrating.* Waco, TX: Word Music, 1986.

"Oliver Wendell Holmes quotes." ThinkExist.com. http://www.thinkexist.com/quotation (accessed August 5, 2011).

"Quote by C.S. Lewis: If you think of this world as a place simply in...." Share Book Recommendations with Your Friends, Join Book Clubs, Answer Trivia. http://www.goodreads.com/quotes/379881-if-you-think-of-this-world-as-a-place-simply (accessed April 21, 2013).

Russell, Arthur J. *God Calling.* New York: Dodd, Mead and Company Inc., 1989.

Smith, Hannah Whitall, and Melvin Easterday Dieter. *God Is Enough.* Longwood, FL: Xulon Press, 2003.

"Welcoming Prayer" Contemplative Outreach Ltd. Silence Solitude Solidarity Service. http://www.contemplativeoutreach.org/category/category/welcoming-prayer (accessed October 1, 2012).

CPSIA information can be obtained at www.ICGtesting.com
Printed in the USA
BVOW08s1645160314

347711BV00002B/43/P

9 781614 489344